ESPAUR Report Webinar and Antibiotic Guardian Shared Learning Awards

ESPAUR Report Webinar and Antibiotic Guardian Shared Learning Awards

Editors

David Enoch
Diane Ashiru-Oredope

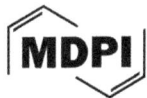

Basel • Beijing • Wuhan • Barcelona • Belgrade • Novi Sad • Cluj • Manchester

Editors
David Enoch
United Kingdom Health
Security Agency (UKHSA)
London
UK

Diane Ashiru-Oredope
United Kingdom Health
Security Agency (UKHSA)
London
UK

Editorial Office
MDPI
St. Alban-Anlage 66
4052 Basel, Switzerland

This is a reprint of articles from the Proceedings published online in the open access journal *Medical Sciences Forum* (ISSN 2673-9992) (available at: https://www.mdpi.com/2673-9992/15/1).

For citation purposes, cite each article independently as indicated on the article page online and as indicated below:

Lastname, A.A.; Lastname, B.B. Article Title. *Journal Name* **Year**, *Volume Number*, Page Range.

ISBN 978-3-7258-0355-2 (Hbk)
ISBN 978-3-7258-0356-9 (PDF)
doi.org/10.3390/books978-3-7258-0356-9

© 2024 by the authors. Articles in this book are Open Access and distributed under the Creative Commons Attribution (CC BY) license. The book as a whole is distributed by MDPI under the terms and conditions of the Creative Commons Attribution-NonCommercial-NoDerivs (CC BY-NC-ND) license.

Contents

About the Editors ix

Neil Cunningham, Ella Casale, Carry Triggs-Hodge, Colin S. Brown, Russell Hope, Diane Ashiru-Oredope and Susan Hopkins
Introduction to the ESPAUR Webinar and Report 2021–2022: Key Findings and Stakeholder Engagement [†]
Reprinted from: *Med. Sci. Forum* **2022**, *15*, 18, doi:10.3390/msf2022015018 1

Rebecca Guy, Hannah Higgins, Jamie Rudman, Holly Fountain, Kirsty F. Bennet, Katie L. Hopkins, et al.
Antimicrobial Resistance in England 2017 to 2021 (ESPAUR Report 2021–2022) [†]
Reprinted from: *Med. Sci. Forum* **2022**, *15*, 3, doi:10.3390/msf2022015003 8

Sabine Bou-Antoun, Angela Falola, Holly Fountain, Hanna Squire, Colin S. Brown, Susan Hopkins, et al.
Antimicrobial Consumption in England, 2017 to 2021 [†]
Reprinted from: *Med. Sci. Forum* **2023**, *15*, 1, doi:10.3390/msf2022015001 13

Kieran Hand, Diane Ashiru-Oredope, Elizabeth Beech, Sabine Bou-Antoun, Gillian Damant, Naomi Fleming, et al.
ESPAUR Report 2021 to 2022 Chapter 5: NHS England Improvement and Assurance Schemes [†]
Reprinted from: *Med. Sci. Forum* **2023**, *15*, 16, doi:10.3390/msf2022015016 19

Ella Casale, Catherine V. Hayes, Donna Lecky, Luke O'Neil, Eirwen Sides, Emily Cooper, et al.
National Antimicrobial Stewardship Activities in Primary and Secondary Care in England 2021–2022 (ESPAUR Report) [†]
Reprinted from: *Med. Sci. Forum* **2023**, *15*, 14, doi:10.3390/msf2022015014 24

Catherine V. Hayes, Jordan Charlesworth, Diane Ashiru-Oredope, Eirwen Sides, Amy Jackson, Emily Cooper, et al.
Antimicrobial Resistance: Professional and Public Education, Engagement, and Training Activities 2021–2022 (ESPAUR Report) [†]
Reprinted from: *Med. Sci. Forum* **2022**, *15*, 19, doi:10.3390/msf2022015019 28

Alessandra Løchen, Hanna Squire, Diane Ashiru-Oredope, Kieran S. Hand, Hassan Hartman, Carry Triggs-Hodge, et al.
Surveillance and Stewardship Approaches for COVID-19 Novel Therapeutics in England from 2021 to 2022 (ESPAUR Report) [†]
Reprinted from: *Med. Sci. Forum* **2022**, *15*, 2, doi:10.3390/msf2022015002 32

Emily Agnew and Julie V. Robotham
Research on Antimicrobial Utilization and Resistance in England 2021–22 (ESPAUR Report) [†]
Reprinted from: *Med. Sci. Forum* **2022**, *15*, 17, doi:10.3390/msf2022015017 37

Fiona Lovatt, Lucy Coyne, Amy Thompson, Georgia Monaghan, Ashley Doorly and Chris Gush
Farm Vet Champion Delivery of Training and SMART Goal Setting to Improve Antimicrobial Stewardship in Farm Veterinary Practice [†]
Reprinted from: *Med. Sci. Forum* **2023**, *15*, 4, doi:10.3390/msf2022015004 43

Balwinder Bolla, Tom Rennison, Catherine Cox, Rupen Tamang, Magda Krupczak and Yui Ka Ho
Supporting Timely IV to Oral Antibiotic Switch through Development of Accessible Clinical Decision Tools †
Reprinted from: *Med. Sci. Forum* **2022**, *15*, 6, doi:10.3390/msf2022015006 . . . . **46**

Grace Biyinzika Lubega, David Musoke, Suzan Nakalawa, Claire Brandish, Bee Yean Ng, Filimin Niyongabo, et al.
Scaling-Up Interventions for Strengthening Antimicrobial Stewardship Using a One Health Approach in Wakiso District, Uganda †
Reprinted from: *Med. Sci. Forum* **2022**, *15*, 7, doi:10.3390/msf2022015007 . . . . **49**

Marta Wanat, Sibyl Anthierens, Marta Santillo, Catherine Porter, Joanne Fielding, Mina Davoudianfar, et al.
Managing Penicillin Allergy in Primary Care: An Important but Neglected Aspect of Antibiotic Stewardship †
Reprinted from: *Med. Sci. Forum* **2022**, *15*, 8, doi:10.3390/msf2022015008 . . . . **53**

William Hope, James Amos, Sarah Atwood, Kyle Bozentko, Amanda Lamb, Gary Leeming, et al.
Informing Antibiotic Guardianship to Combat Antimicrobial Resistance: The Liverpool Citizens' Jury on AMR †
Reprinted from: *Med. Sci. Forum* **2022**, *15*, 9, doi:10.3390/msf2022015009 . . . . **56**

Sarah Cavanagh, Frances Garraghan, Maxencia Nabiryo, Diane Ashiru-Oredope, Melvin Bell and Victoria Rutter
Developing a Board and Online Game to Educate People on Antimicrobial Resistance and Stewardship: The AMS Game †
Reprinted from: *Med. Sci. Forum* **2022**, *15*, 12, doi:10.3390/msf2022015012 . . . . **60**

Paula Anabalon-Cordova, Susie Sanderson, David Williams, Mahesh Verma, Céline Pulcini, Leanne Teoh and Wendy Thompson
Engaging the Global Dental Profession to Help Tackle Antibiotic Resistance †
Reprinted from: *Med. Sci. Forum* **2022**, *15*, 13, doi:10.3390/msf2022015013 . . . . **62**

Balwinder Bolla and Alex Rond-Alliston
Supporting Correct Antimicrobial Choices in Sepsis †
Reprinted from: *Med. Sci. Forum* **2022**, *15*, 5, doi:10.3390/msf2022015005 . . . . **66**

Rakhi Aggarwal, Angela Barker, Conor Jamieson and Donna Cooper
Antibiotic Amnesty: Engaging with the Public across the Midlands Region of England †
Reprinted from: *Med. Sci. Forum* **2022**, *15*, 10, doi:10.3390/msf2022015010 . . . . **69**

Shima Chundoo, Conor Jamieson, Rob Tobin and Anna Hunt
Dental Antimicrobial Prescribing in the Midlands: A Regional Action Plan †
Reprinted from: *Med. Sci. Forum* **2022**, *15*, 11, doi:10.3390/msf2022015011 . . . . **72**

Jessica Fraser, Frances Garraghan and Diane Ashiru-Oredope
Development and User Feedback on Antimicrobial Stewardship Explainer Videos: A Collaborative Approach between the UK and Eight African Countries †
Reprinted from: *Med. Sci. Forum* **2022**, *15*, 15, doi:10.3390/msf2022015015 . . . . **77**

Michael Mosha, Erick Venant, Baltazari Stanley, Fatuma Denis, Dorinegrace Mushi, Eva Ombaka and Karin Wiedenmayer
Schoolchildren as Agents of Change towards Antimicrobial Resistance †
Reprinted from: *Med. Sci. Forum* **2023**, *15*, 20, doi:10.3390/msf2022015020 . . . . **81**

Diane Ashiru-Oredope, Carry Triggs-Hodge and Jordan Charlesworth
Statement of Peer Review [†]
Reprinted from: *Med. Sci. Forum* **2023**, *15*, 21, doi:10.3390/msf2022015021 . . . . **84**

About the Editors

David Enoch

Dr. David Enoch is a consultant microbiologist with the UK Health Security Agency and Cambridge University Hospitals NHS Foundation Trust. He trained in medicine at St Bartholomew's Hospital in London and worked in the fields of infectious diseases and HIV medicine in Ealing and the Royal Free Hospitals in London before moving to Cambridge as a microbiology registrar. His first consultant post was in Peterborough, before he returned to Cambridge in 2013. His interests include healthcare-associated infections and invasive fungal infections/antifungal stewardship.

Diane Ashiru-Oredope

Professor Diane Ashiru-Oredope is the Lead Pharmacist for the Antimicrobial Resistance and Healthcare Associated Infections, UK Health Security Agency, and Honorary Chair and Professor of Pharmaceutical Public Health at the University of Nottingham. An antimicrobial pharmacist by background, she chairs the English Surveillance Programme for Antimicrobial Utilisation and Resistance (ESPAUR), the National Planning Group for World Antimicrobial Awareness activities in England, and the UK Antibiotic Guardian campaign.

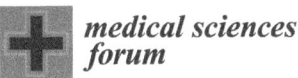

Editorial

Introduction to the ESPAUR Webinar and Report 2021–2022: Key Findings and Stakeholder Engagement [†]

Neil Cunningham, Ella Casale, Carry Triggs-Hodge, Colin S. Brown, Russell Hope, Diane Ashiru-Oredope * and Susan Hopkins

HCAI, Fungal, AMR, AMU & Sepsis Division, United Kingdom Health Security Agency (UKHSA), London NW9 5EQ, UK; neil.cunningham@ukhsa.gov.uk (N.C.); carry.triggshodge@ukhsa.gov.uk (C.T.-H.)
* Correspondence: diane.ashiru-oredope@ukhsa.gov.uk
† Presented at the ESPAUR 2021/22 Webinar, Antibiotic Guardian, 23 November 2022; Available online: https://antibioticguardian.com/Meetings/espaur-2021-22-webinar/.

Abstract: During the coronavirus (COVID-19) pandemic, we saw significant decreases in the incidence of bloodstream infections (BSIs), antibiotic-resistant infections, and the burden of resistant infections. The reasons for this are complex and multifactorial, but likely, at least in part, due to changes in healthcare delivery and healthcare seeking behavior. As healthcare systems return to pre-pandemic ways of working, now is a pivotal moment to ensure focus remains on what is often referred to as the 'silent pandemic': antimicrobial resistance (AMR). The ninth English Surveillance Programme for Antimicrobial Utilization and Resistance (ESPAUR) report provides an overview of the national data on antibiotic prescribing and resistance, antimicrobial stewardship implementation, and awareness activities. The active contribution from and collaboration with the ESPAUR oversight group and the engagement of stakeholder organizations, including the devolved administrations, are also reported. Findings from the ESPAUR report were presented at a webinar on 23 November 2022.

Keywords: antimicrobial consumption; antimicrobial resistance; antimicrobial stewardship; antibiotic; anti-fungal; England

Citation: Cunningham, N.; Casale, E.; Triggs-Hodge, C.; Brown, C.S.; Hope, R.; Ashiru-Oredope, D.; Hopkins, S. Introduction to the ESPAUR Webinar and Report 2021–2022: Key Findings and Stakeholder Engagement. *Med. Sci. Forum* **2022**, *15*, 18. https://doi.org/10.3390/msf2022015018

Published: 8 May 2023

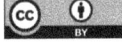

Copyright: © 2023 by the authors. Licensee MDPI, Basel, Switzerland. This article is an open access article distributed under the terms and conditions of the Creative Commons Attribution (CC BY) license (https://creativecommons.org/licenses/by/4.0/).

1. Introduction

Findings from the English Surveillance Programme for Antimicrobial Utilization and Resistance (ESPAUR) report were presented at the ESPAUR 2021/22 webinar. UKHSA hosted the ESPAUR 2021–22 report interactive webinar on Wednesday 23 November 2022. The recording is available.

ESPAUR was established by the UK Health Security Agency (UKHSA) in 2013 to support the delivery of the UK National Action Plan (NAP) for antimicrobial resistance (AMR) [1]. The ESPAUR programme and oversight group works across the healthcare system, and with external stakeholders to bring together the elements of antimicrobial utilization and resistance surveillance to inform on trends and the impact of external forces on antimicrobial prescribing, and progress towards the 5-year NAP.

The aims of ESPAUR are to (1) develop and maintain robust surveillance systems for monitoring and reporting trends in antimicrobial use and resistance, in order to measure the impact of surveillance, antimicrobial stewardship, and other interventions on antimicrobial resistance that affect human health, and (2) develop systems and processes to optimize antimicrobial prescribing across healthcare settings [2].

Chapter 1 of the ESPAUR report provides an overview of the key messages from each chapter [3] (Figure 1). Data and data sources, data processing and statistical analyses are detailed in the ESPAUR Report Annexe [4].

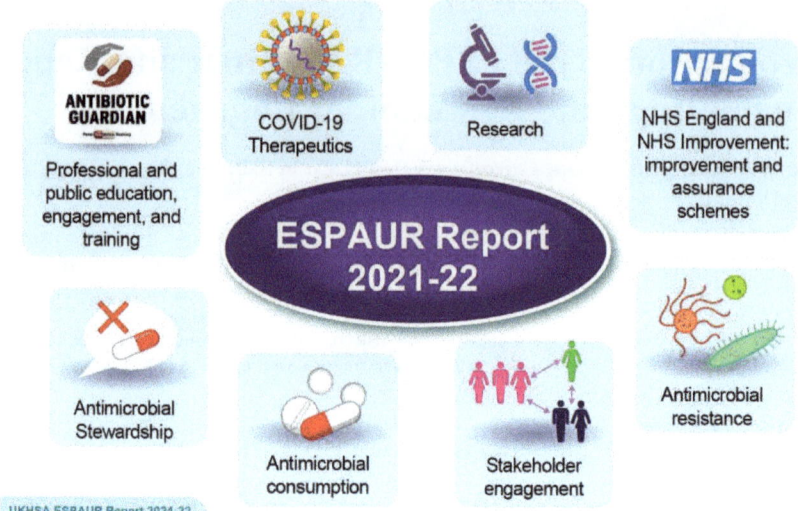

Figure 1. Chapters in the ESPAUR report 2021–2022. Reprinted with permission from Ref. [4]. Copyright 2022 UK Health Security Agency.

2. Highlights from the Chapters

2.1. Chapter 2—Antimicrobial Resistance (AMR)

The UK NAP ambition for AMR is to reduce the (estimated) total number of antibiotic-resistant infections in the UK by 10% from the 2018 baseline by 2025 [5]. Progress has been made towards this target, with a 9.1% reduction being achieved between 2018 and 2021 in England, although much of this reduction occurred during the pandemic and is likely to be in part due to the interventions in place at that time [6]. After an initial increase seen between 2018 and 2019, there was a 15.7% decline in the estimated number of severe antibiotic-resistant infections between 2019 and 2020, followed by a slight increase in 2021 (2.2%) [6].

For the first time in the ESPAUR report, data have been disaggregated to describe varying rates of AMR burden related to ethnicity and deprivation. The rate of carbapenems-producing Gram-negative bacteria notifications varied by indices of multiple deprivation (IMD), with a higher rate of notifications seen in the more deprived deciles (2021: 6.8 per 100,000 population in the most deprived decile compared with 2.8 per 100,000 population in the least deprived) [6]. In 2021, 81% (50,329) of BSI episodes (as per AMR burden combinations) were recorded in persons within a white ethnic group, of which 20.9% were resistant to at least one key antimicrobial [6]. The highest percentage resistance was noted in the Asian or Asian British ethnic group, with 32.8% of key organisms BSI-resistant to at least one key antimicrobial [6]. Further work to develop a deeper understanding of the impact of ethnicity, deprivation, regional divergence, along with potential confounders, remains a crucial avenue of enquiry and essential to the identification of appropriate target interventions. UKHSA has developed an AMR health inequalities workstream to better understand how the burden of AMR differentially impacts certain groups, and to embed a systematic approach to reducing health inequalities in AMR.

2.2. Chapter 3—Antimicrobial Consumption

Total antibiotic consumption has been decreasing with a sharp decline seen coinciding with the COVID-19 pandemic. There was an overall 10.9% decrease in antibiotic consumption between 2019 and 2020 alone, followed by a further decline of 0.5% from 2020 to 2021 [7]. Antibiotic prescribing continued to be the highest in the general practice setting in 2021 (72.1%) and it is also here that the largest reductions in antibiotic prescribing have consistently occurred [7]. In 2021, antibiotic prescribing has also decreased in dental practices, following a spike between 2019 and 2020, but has increased in hospital inpatient, outpatient, and other community settings between 2020 and 2021 [7].

Total consumption of systemic antifungals prescribed in the community and NHS hospitals in England decreased by 22.9% between 2017 and 2021. However, between 2020 and 2021, antifungal consumption has increased by 7.1% [7].

The reasons for the fall in antimicrobial consumption are likely multifactorial, but driven by a reduction in respiratory infections, supported by reports of reduced respiratory antibiotic prescribing in the young [8], and reduced general practice consultations [9]. Other factors likely include improved infection prevention and control measures, social restrictions, the use of facemasks, and changes in-service delivery, such as less face-to-face consultations in primary care.

2.3. Chapter 4—Antimicrobial Stewardship

Whilst improvements and reductions in antibiotic prescribing have been made, continued stewardship and surveillance are needed to sustain progress towards the NAP. The factors contributing to improvements in antimicrobial stewardship are likely multifactorial, but UKHSA continues to lead some of the key national primary and secondary care antimicrobial stewardship (AMS) interventions, including the TARGET (Treat Antibiotics Responsibly, Guidance, Education and Tools) toolkit hosted on the Royal College of General Practitioners (RCGP) website [10], and Start Smart then Focus (AMS toolkit for secondary care).

The TARGET Antibiotic Checklist [11], an antimicrobial stewardship tool, was included as a component of the 2021 to 2022 Pharmacy Quality Scheme (PQS), and 74% of pharmacies in England submitted data from over 200,000 individuals collecting an antibiotic prescription. High engagement from pharmacy staff suggests that the AMS principles introduced with the TARGET Antibiotic Checklist may be embedded [12].

In line with the NAP ambition to "enhance the role of pharmacists in primary care", UKHSA, in collaboration with partners, has developed evidence-based, system-wide intervention ('How to...' guides) to support primary care teams to review the dose and duration of long-term and repeat antimicrobial prescriptions. The intervention focuses on toolkits and resource guides, specifically for acne and chronic obstructive pulmonary disease exacerbations (COPD). Acne and COPD were prioritized as Primary Care Network (PCN) data, revealing that these are the most common clinical conditions associated with the highest use of long-term or repeat antibiotics [12].

Within secondary care, AMS interventions included the development of a UK-wide antimicrobial intravenous-to-oral switch (IVOS) criteria and sample tools for hospitalised adult patients. This was developed from local policies, literature, and expert opinion with consensus for switch criteria obtained via a 4-stage Delphi process involving 279 multidisciplinary colleagues from all four UK nations [12].

2.4. Chapter 5—NHS England: Improvement and Assurance Schemes

Within primary care, the NHS System Oversight Framework 2021/22, which aims to ensure alignment of priorities across the NHS, retained two primary care antibiotic prescribing metrics: total items prescribed and broad-spectrum proportion [13]. By the end of 2021 to 2022, 50% of 42 Integrated Care Systems (ICSs: local partnerships of NHS providers, local authorities, and others who have collective responsibility for planning services, improving health and reducing inequalities for their population of 500,000 to 3 million) met the NAP reduction target for total antibiotic prescribing and 83% met the reduction target for the proportion of broad-spectrum antibiotics [9].

For NHS trusts providing acute care, a requirement to reduce antibiotic consumption by 2% from each trust's 2018 calendar year baseline was reinstated in the NHS Standard Contract for 2021 to 2022, following suspension during the COVID-19 pandemic [14]. By the end of 2021 to 2022, 50% of acute trusts met this ambition to reduce a total consumption of antimicrobials by 2% [9].

2.5. Chapter 6—Professional and Public Education, Engagement and Training

UKHSA continues to lead the education and engagement of healthcare professionals and the public through World Antimicrobial Awareness Week (WAAW), European Antibiotic Awareness Day (EAAD), and the National Healthcare Students' AMR Conference for medical and pharmacy students.

WAAW 2021 offered an opportunity to engage professionals and the public in AMR by consolidating digital campaigning introduced in 2020. A new WAAW and EAAD toolkit for healthcare professionals in England was developed to provide guidance to support the NHS, local authorities and others to lead activities and encourage the responsible use of antibiotics. There was also continued engagement with Antibiotic Guardian Schools Ambassadors providing antibiotic use, and infection prevention and control education to children and young people through schools and community groups [15].

A redesign and national rollout of the e-Bug resources is helping meet objectives to support schools and communities to reinvigorate key infection prevention and control (IPC), and AMR messages [16]. Groundwork for the national implementation of TARGET and e-Bug professional training and resources has commenced, aiming for consistent education of healthcare professionals (HCP) and the public in the future [15].

2.6. Chapter 7—COVID-19 Therapeutics

UKHSA's COVID-19 therapeutics programme has supported the deployment of COVID-19 therapies by undertaking genomic, virological, and epidemiological surveillance of COVID-19 therapeutics. Between 1 October 2021 and 31 March 2022, there were over 51,000 treatment requests for neutralizing monoclonal antibodies and antivirals against COVID-19 for patients in England [17]. This programme identified eleven mutations which exhibited a significant change between samples obtained from patients before and after treatment, and which may help the virus evade antimicrobials. This has been an important evidence base for changes to clinical commissioning policies for COVID-19 therapeutics [18].

2.7. Chapter 8—Research

The UKHSA continues to undertake a wide range of new and ongoing research projects in the field of healthcare-associated infections (HCAIs) and AMR, which cover many of the major themes of the NAP for AMR. Key research is presented from the two National Institute for Health Research (NIHR) Health Protection Research Units (HPRUs), led by the Imperial College London and Oxford University in partnership with UKHSA. The research outputs are described in further detail in Chapter 8 of the ESPAUR Report [19].

3. Stakeholder Engagement

UKHSA could not deliver its range of activities, progress towards its objectives or produce the ESPAUR report without active contribution from and collaboration with the ESPAUR oversight group and the engagement of stakeholder organizations (Figure 2). More than 20 national stakeholders, ranging from government organizations to independent healthcare providers to patient representatives, are current and active members of the ESPAUR Oversight Group and contribute to reducing AMR in the United Kingdom:

- Department of Health and Social Care (DHSC), including Dental Public Health, Office for Health Improvement and Disparities (OHID)
- DHSC Expert Advisory Committee on Antimicrobial Prescribing, Resistance and Healthcare-Associated Infection (APRHAI)
- British National Formulary (BNF)
- British Society for Antimicrobial Chemotherapy (BSAC)
- Care Quality Commission (CQC)

- College of General Dentistry
- IQVIA
- National Institute of Health and Care Excellence (NICE)
- NHS England (NHSE)
- Patient representation
- Primary Care Pharmacy Association (PCPA)
- Royal College of Nursing (RCN)
- Royal College of Physicians (RCP)
- Royal College of General Practitioners (RCGP)
- Royal Pharmaceutical Society (RPS)
- Rx-Info Ltd.
- UK Clinical Pharmacy Association: Pharmacy Infection Network (UKCPA PIN)
- Veterinary Medicines Directorate (DEFRA)
- Antimicrobial Resistance and Healthcare-Associated Infection (ARHAI) Scotland, NHS National Services Scotland
- Public Health Scotland
- Public Health Wales
- Public Health Agency Northern Ireland (Health and Social Care Northern Ireland-HSCNI)
- UKHSA (represented by individuals with appropriate expertise from the HCAI, antimicrobial utilization (AMU), AMR, Fungal and Sepsis Division, Behavioral Insights, Regions, Field Service, Microbiology services, and Communications teams)

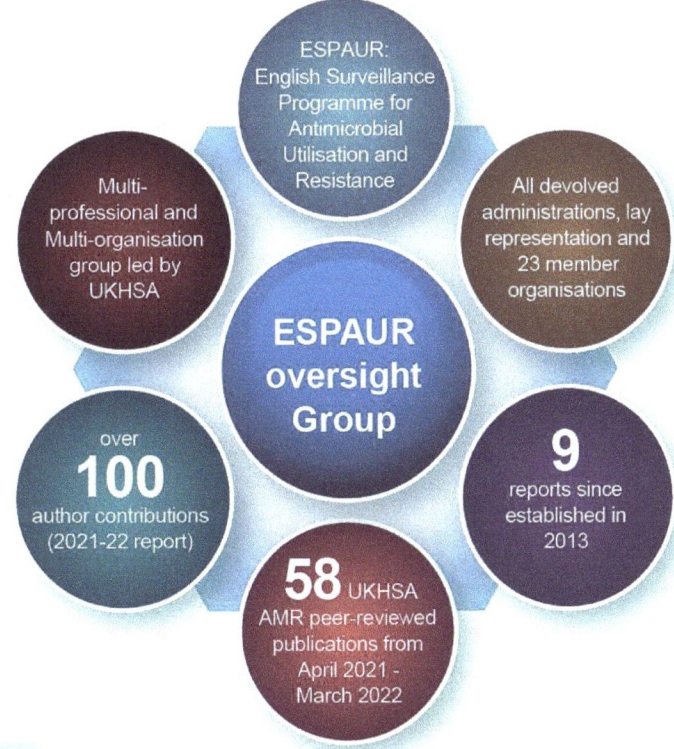

Figure 2. Key outputs of the ESPAUR oversight group. Reprinted with permission from Ref. [4]. Copyright 2022 UK Health Security Agency.

Stakeholder Activities

A wide range of stakeholder activities have been undertaken over the previous year. The following activity is an example of the range of stakeholder undertakings with the aim of reducing AMR: resources, such as the TARGET Antibiotics toolkit [3], have been promoted across the UK via the use of campaigns and other methods. One such campaign, run in 2021, aimed to introduce the 'Antibiotic Checklist', including a resource pack with self-care leaflets and posters, to all community pharmacies in Wales.

Furthermore, there has been significant commitment over the previous year to develop educational resources, publish evidence-based resources, and promote AMS programmes. For example, to facilitate the use of the Antibiotic Checklist, an E-Learning module was developed in collaboration with stakeholders involved in health education and improvement. This module was based on the E-Learning module previously developed by PHE (now UKHSA) and Health Education England. Pharmacy stakeholders have also developed a range of pharmacy resources, including podcasts, blogs, and webinars, and an education programme on infection prevention and control and antimicrobial stewardship, using competencies developed with the University of Cardiff, has continued to be delivered.

In addition to these activities, the ESPAUR Oversight Group has provided support to national and international networks by contributing to the European Antibiotic Awareness Day and World Health Organization's Antimicrobial Awareness Week. For example, public health colleagues ran a campaign during WAAW 2021 to highlight the importance of AMR to both professionals and the public. Finally, the surveillance of AMR infections has been improved following the launch of the NHS AMR dashboard. This allows key data on emergency admissions due to bacterial infection and/or sepsis to be viewed at the Integrated Care System, Clinical Commissioning Group, NHS Trust, and regional and national levels, broken down by individual criteria.

Author Contributions: Conceptualization, D.A.-O. and S.H.; methodology, N.C., E.C. and C.T.-H.; validation, C.S.B. and R.H.; resources, D.A.-O., C.S.B., R.H. and S.H.; writing—original draft preparation, N.C., E.C. and C.T.-H.; visualization, E.C. and C.T.-H.; project administration, E.C. and C.T.-H. All authors have read and agreed to the published version of the manuscript.

Funding: This editorial received no external funding.

Institutional Review Board Statement: Not applicable.

Informed Consent Statement: Not applicable.

Data Availability Statement: Publicly available datasets were analyzed in this study. This data can be found here: English surveillance programme for antimicrobial utilization and resistance (ESPAUR) report—GOV.UK (www.gov.uk, accessed on 25 November 2022).

Acknowledgments: The authors would like to acknowledge the ESPAUR Oversight Group members and individual chapter authors for their dedication and contribution. Contributors to the stakeholder chapter are also acknowledged: Gil Damant, Tamsin Dewe, Jeff Featherstone, Kitty Healey, Martin Astbury, Natasha Bell-Asher, Nicholas Brown, Mary Collier, Judith Ewing, Naomi Fleming, Rose Gallagher, Ellie Gillham, Kieran Hand, Martin Llewelyn, William Malcolm, Sannah Malik, Arianne Matlin, Nicholas Reid, Tracy Rogers, Wendy Thompson, Jonathan Underhill, Fiona Watson, Lydia Harman, and Simon Hartnett-Welch.

Conflicts of Interest: The authors declare no conflict of interest.

References

1. *Tackling Antimicrobial Resistance 2019 to 2024: The UK's 5-Year National Action Plan*; Department of Health and Social Care: London, UK, 2019.
2. Hopkins, S.; Johnson, A. Chapter 1 Introduction. In *The English Surveillance Programme for Antimicrobial Utilisation and Resistance (ESPAUR) Report 2018*; Public Health England: London, UK, 2018.
3. Cunningham, N.; Hopkins, S. Chapter 1 Introduction. In *The English Surveillance Programme for Antimicrobial Utilisation and Resistance (ESPAUR) Report 2021 to 2022*; UK Health Security Agency: London, UK, 2022.

4. UK Health Security Agency. English surveillance programme for antimicrobial utilisation and resistance (ESPAUR) Report 2021 to 2022. Available online: https://www.gov.uk/government/publications/english-surveillance-programme-antimicrobial-utilisation-and-resistance-espaur-report (accessed on 25 November 2022).
5. *Tackling Antimicrobial Resistance 2019 to 2024: Addendum to the UK's 5-Year National Action Plan*; Department of Health and Social Care: London, UK, 2022.
6. Guy, R.; Higgins, H.; Rudman, J.; Fountain, H.; Henderson, K.; Bennet, K.; Hopkins, K.; Demirjian, A.; Gerver, S.; Mirfenderesky, M. Chapter 2 Antimicrobial Resistance. In *The English Surveillance Programme for Antimicrobial Utilisation and Resistance (ESPAUR) Report 2021-22*; UK Health Security Agency: London, UK, 2022.
7. Bou-Antoun, S.; Falola, A.; Fountain, H.; Squire, H.; Brown, C.; Hopkins, S.; Gerver, S.; Demirjian, A. Chapter 3 Antimicrobial consumption. In *The English Surveillance Programme for Antimicrobial Utilisation and Resistance (ESPAUR) Report 2021 to 2022*; UK Health Security Agency: London, UK, 2022.
8. Andrews, A.; Bou-Antoun, S.; Guy, R.; Brown, C.S.; Hopkins, S.; Gerver, S. Respiratory antibacterial prescribing in primary care and the COVID-19 pandemic in England, winter season 2020–21. *J. Antimicrob. Chemother.* **2022**, *77*, 799–802. [CrossRef] [PubMed]
9. Hand, K.; Beech, E.; McLeod, M.; Bou-Antoun, S.; Squire, H.; Budd, E.; Featherstone, J.; Parekh, S.; Lecky, D.; Hayes, C.; et al. Chapter 5 NHS England: Improvement and assurance schemes. In *The English Surveillance Programme for Antimicrobial Utilisation and Resistance (ESPAUR) Report 2021 to 2022*; UK Health Security Agency: London, UK, 2022.
10. Royal College of General Practitioners. TARGET Antibiotics Toolkit Hub. 2022. Available online: https://elearning.rcgp.org.uk/course/view.php?id=553 (accessed on 25 November 2022).
11. Royal College of General Practitioners. TARGET Antibiotics Toolkit Hub—TARGET Antibiotic Checklist. 2022. Available online: https://elearning.rcgp.org.uk/mod/book/view.php?id=13511&chapterid=784 (accessed on 25 November 2022).
12. Casale, E.; Hayes, C.; Lecky, D.; O'Neil, L.; Sides, E.; Cooper, E.; Pursey, F.; Parekh, S.; Fisher, L.; MacKenna, B.; et al. Chapter 4 Antimicrobial stewardship. In *The English Surveillance Programme for Antimicrobial Utilisation and Resistance (ESPAUR) Report 2021 to 2022*; UK Health Security Agency: London, UK, 2022.
13. NHS England. NHS System Oversight Framework 2021/22. 2021. Available online: https://www.england.nhs.uk/publication/system-oversight-framework-2021-22/ (accessed on 25 November 2022).
14. NHS England. 2021/22 NHS Standard Contract. 2021. Available online: https://www.england.nhs.uk/nhs-standard-contract/previous-nhs-standard-contracts/21-22/ (accessed on 25 November 2022).
15. Hayes, C.; Charlesworth, J.; Ashiru-Oredope, D.; Sides, E.; Jackson, A.; Cooper, E.; Read, B.; Seaton, D.; Flintham, L.; Sidhu, H.; et al. Chapter 6 Professional education and training and public engagement. In *The English Surveillance Programme for Antimicrobial Utilisation and Resistance (ESPAUR) Report 2021 to 2022*; UK Health Security Agency: London, UK, 2022.
16. e-Bug. 2022. Available online: https://e-Bug.eu (accessed on 25 November 2022).
17. Squire, H.; Lochen, A.; Ashiru-Oredope, D.; Hand, K.; Hartman, H.; Triggs-Hodge, C.; Fountain, H.; Bou-Antoun, S.; Gerver, S.; Demirjian, A. Chapter 7. COVID-19 therapeutics. In *The English Surveillance Programme for Antimicrobial Utilisation and Resistance (ESPAUR) Report 2021 to 2022*; UK Health Security Agency: London, UK, 2022.
18. UK Health Security Agency. COVID-19 Therapeutic Agents: Technical Briefings. 2022. Available online: https://www.gov.uk/government/publications/covid-19-therapeutic-agents-technical-briefings (accessed on 25 November 2022).
19. Agnew, E.; Charlesworth, J.; Bacon, J.; Charani, E.; Turton, J.; Guy, R.; Lipworth, S.; Borek, A.; Collin, S.; Ashiru-Oredope, D.; et al. Chapter 8 Research. In *The English Surveillance Programme for Antimicrobial Utilisation and Resistance (ESPAUR) Report 2021 to 2022*; UK Health Security Agency: London, UK, 2022.

Disclaimer/Publisher's Note: The statements, opinions and data contained in all publications are solely those of the individual author(s) and contributor(s) and not of MDPI and/or the editor(s). MDPI and/or the editor(s) disclaim responsibility for any injury to people or property resulting from any ideas, methods, instructions or products referred to in the content.

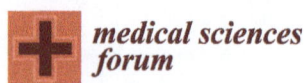

Proceeding Paper

Antimicrobial Resistance in England 2017 to 2021 (ESPAUR Report 2021–2022) †

Rebecca Guy [1,*], Hannah Higgins [1], Jamie Rudman [1], Holly Fountain [1], Kirsty F. Bennet [1], Katie L. Hopkins [1], Alicia Demirjian [1,2,3], Sarah M. Gerver [1], Mariyam Mirfenderesky [1,4] and Katherine L. Henderson [1,*]

1. Healthcare-Associated Infections, Fungal, Antimicrobial Resistance, Antimicrobial Usage and Sepsis Division, United Kingdom Health Security Agency (UKHSA), London NW9 5EQ, UK
2. Department of Paediatric Infectious Diseases & Immunology, Evelina London Children's Hospital, London SE1 7EH, UK
3. Faculty of Life Sciences & Medicine, King's College London, London WC2R 2LS, UK
4. Microbiology Department, North Middlesex University Hospital NHS Trust, London N18 1QX, UK
* Correspondence: rebecca.guy@ukhsa.gov.uk (R.G.); katherine.henderson@ukhsa.gov.uk (K.L.H.)
† Presented at the ESPAUR 2021/22 Webinar, Antibiotic Guardian, 23 November 2022; Available online: https://antibioticguardian.com/Meetings/espaur-2021-22-webinar/.

Abstract: The English surveillance programme for antimicrobial utilisation and resistance (ESPAUR) antimicrobial resistance (AMR) chapter reports on bacterial, viral, and fungal AMR trends between 2017 and 2021 in England. A 10.8% increase in patient episodes of bacteraemia or fungaemia was observed, and the estimated burden of resistance decreased by 4.2%. Individuals with an antimicrobial-resistant strain (resistant to ≥1 key AMR burden-defined antibiotics) had a higher crude case fatality rate (18.1%) compared to those with a susceptible strain (16.3%). The effect of deprivation on carbapenemase-producing organisms (CPO) incidence, and the impact of the AMR burden across ethnic groups, have been described for the first time. Understanding the impact of ethnicity, deprivation, regional divergence, and potential confounders remains a crucial avenue of enquiry to target appropriate AMR interventions. These findings were presented at the ESPAUR Report webinar on 23 November 2022.

Keywords: antimicrobial; resistance; England; bacterial; fungal; viral; AMR; ethnicity; deprivation; health inequality

1. Introduction

Antibiotic resistance is an increasing, established threat to global health, with an estimated 4.9 million associated deaths recorded in 2019 globally [1] and simple surgeries becoming more dangerous due to lack of effective antibiotics [2]. The UK Government has committed to a 5- and 20-year vision to reduce antimicrobial resistance (AMR) [3,4], with a national action plan (NAP) for monitoring progress. The English surveillance programme for antimicrobial utilisation and resistance (ESPAUR) report AMR chapter reports on key AMR trends [5,6].

2. Methods

2.1. Data and Data Sources

Bloodstream infections (BSI) caused by key pathogens were taken from routine and reference laboratory data for England for 2017–2021 [5]. Key pathogens included the Gram-negative bacteria: *Escherichia coli*, *Klebsiella pneumoniae*, *Klebsiella oxytoca*, *Pseudomonas* spp., and *Acinetobacter* spp.; and Gram-positive bacteria: *Enterococcus faecalis*, *Enterococcus faecium*, *Staphylococcus aureus* group, and *Streptococcus pneumoniae*. The carbapenemase-producing Gram-negative bacteria notifications were extracted for 2021 only.

The Gram-negative bacteria were reviewed for susceptibility to each of the following: gentamicin, ciprofloxacin, piperacillin/tazobactam, co-amoxiclav, third-generation cephalosporins (cefotaxime, ceftazidime, ceftriaxone, or cefpodoxime; as applicable) and carbapenems (meropenem, imipenem, or ertapenem, as applicable). The Gram-positive bacteria were reviewed for susceptibility to the following: glycopeptides (vancomycin or teicoplanin), penicillin, macrolides (erythromycin, azithromycin, or clarithromycin), and meticillin (flucloxacillin, oxacillin, or cefoxitin).

Susceptibility reports are given as S (susceptible), I (intermediate; susceptible increased exposure), and R (resistant), as recorded by the local laboratory. The samples were deduplicated for patients who had more than one blood culture taken (yielding growth of the same pathogen) during a rolling 14-day period from the initial positive blood culture. Where differing susceptibility results were reported, the worst-case scenario susceptibility result was retained, and, for analysis on resistance, S and I were grouped together.

2.2. Data Processing

The burden of resistant infections is a hierarchical measure adapted from the Cassini et al. method [6] and used in publications within England [5]; it incorporates critical treatment antibiotics in key Gram-negative and -positive infections (see ESPAUR report). Ethnicity data were obtained via linkage to NHS Digital's Hospital Episode Statistic (HES) admission data, following the method outlined by the Office for Health Improvement and Disparities [7]. In addition, Index of Multiple Deprivation (IMD) data from the Office for National Statistics (ONS) were linked to the CPO patients' residential postcodes and were analysed by the IMD decile (1 = most deprived; 10 = least deprived) [5].

2.3. Statistical Analyses

Case fatality rates (CFRs) were calculated and stratified by the specimen group and resistance status, using patients successfully matched to the NHS Spine as the denominator. The CFRs were calculated as the percentage of patients who died with or without an antibiotic-resistant infection relative to the total patients in those groups who had been NHS Spine (NHS Digital)-matched. p-values were calculated to assess the change in resistance over time; these were generated using an unadjusted binomial regression model with a significant change being defined by $p < 0.05$. Incidence rates were calculated per 100,000 population per year using ONS mid-year populations [5]. Exact binomial 95% confidence intervals were calculated for the percentage resistance for the ethnic group analysis. STATA (version 17; StataCorp, Texas, USA) statistical software was used for this analysis.

3. Results

3.1. The Burden of AMR

There was a 10.8% increase in patient episodes of bacteraemia or fungaemia reported from laboratories in England between 2017 (n = 138,417) and 2021 (n = 153,362), of which 88.9% were monomicrobial in 2021, contrasting with a decrease in overall annual total blood cultures reported across this period [8]. For many of the key pathogens reviewed, the incidence of BSI showed an increase between 2017 and 2021 (*K. pneumoniae* (12.0/100,000 population to 13.5), *Pseudomonas* spp. (8.0 to 8.5), *Acinetobacter* spp. (1.6 to 1.8), and *Enterococcus* spp. (12.4 to 15.8)). Over the same time frame, the incidence of *E. coli* and *S. pneumoniae* BSI decreased (74.3/100,000 population to 66.9 and 8.7 to 4.0, respectively), predominantly in 2020 and 2021.

The burden of AMR decreased by 4.2% between 2017 (n = 16,099) and 2021 (n = 15,446; $p = 0.101$; Figure 1). The burden of antibiotic-resistant BSI predominates within the Enterobacterales family (particularly *E. coli*, of which 40% are resistant to the commonly used co-amoxiclav, and 10% are resistant to piperacillin with tazobactam), comprising 80.3% of the total episodes (with the peak in 2019 at 84.8%). The burden of resistant infections remained relatively unchanged between 2017 and 2021 for Gram-positive infections, although an increase of 2.5% in glycopeptide-resistant *Enterococcus* spp. was recorded ($p < 0.0001$).

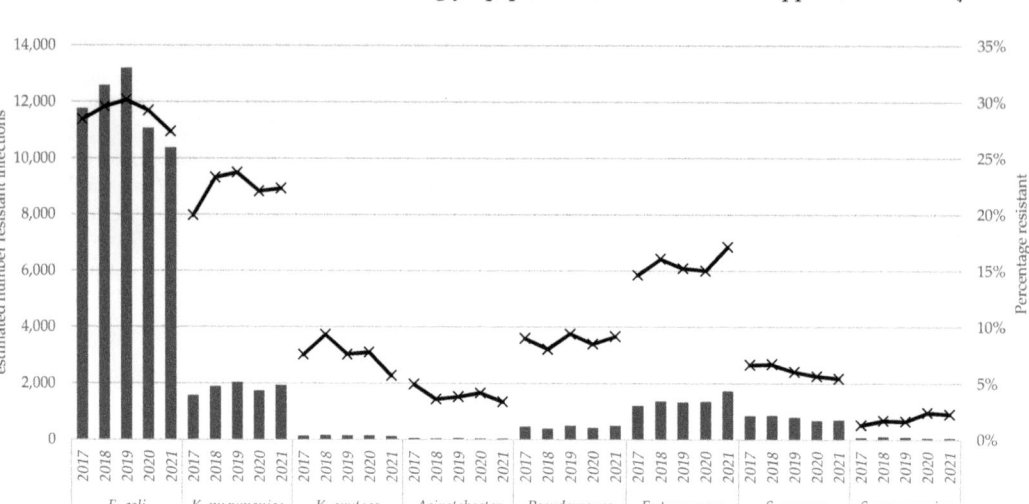

Figure 1. Annual estimated total (of the burden) of antibiotic-resistant bloodstream episodes by species (bar chart, left y-axis) and percentage resistant (line chart, right y-axis); England 2017 to 2021.

The burden of AMR BSI varied by ethnic group. In 2021, the highest number of BSI episodes was recorded in persons within a White ethnic group (80.8%; n = 50,329), of which 20.9% were recorded as resistant to at least one key antimicrobial. Aside from the mix of patients within the 'any other ethnic group' (n = 322; 34.0%), the highest percentage resistance was noted in the 'Asian or Asian British' ethnic group (n = 1243; 32.8%).

The London region reported the highest rate per 100,000 population burden of resistance (55.5/100,000), followed by the North West (44.5) and South East (41.1). The lowest was recorded in the East Midlands (32.1). For the overall incidence of key BSI pathogens, the lowest estimated rate was recorded in the East of England (130.7) and London regions (131.2). The highest rate of key species BSI infection was recorded in the North East (176.5).

When expanded to estimate the number of resistant infections including other infection types (surgical-site infections, urinary tract, and skin/soft-tissue infections), the number of serious antibiotic-resistant infections in England rose by 2.2% in 2021 compared to 2020 (53,985 compared to 52,842; $p < 0.01$), equivalent to 148 severe antibiotic-resistant infections a day in 2021.

3.2. Acquired Carbapenemase-Producing Gram-Negative Bacteria

In 2021, the most frequent carbapenemase family recorded in England was OXA-48-like (915/2244; 40.8%), followed by NDM (563/2244; 25.1%) and KPC (550/2244; 24.5%). In 2021, London and the North West regions reported the largest number of CPOs; however, there is considerable regional variation in both the number and families of carbapenemase being recorded. In the most deprived IMD decile, the rate of CPO notifications was 6.8 per 100,000 population, compared with 2.8 per 100,000 population in the least deprived. The carbapenemase family identified also varied with deprivation; however, the differences may be a result of regional mechanism variations, local screening policies, and outbreaks.

3.3. Thirty-Day All-Cause Mortality

The overall 30-day all-cause CFR in patients with key Gram-negative bacterial BSI (*Escherichia* spp., *Klebsiella* spp., *Pseudomonas* spp., *Acinetobacter* spp.) was 16.7% in 2021 (n = 7627); the CFR was lowest in children aged 1 to 14 years (1.9%, n = 11) and highest in adults aged 85 years and over (21.8%, n = 2053). Individuals with a resistant strain (resistant to ≥ 1 key AMR burden-defined antibiotics) had a higher crude CFR (18.1%, n = 1725; $p < 0.05$) compared to those with a susceptible strain (16.3%, n = 5818). In 2021, the crude 30-day all-cause CFR in people with an invasive CPO was 24.5% (n = 25/102).

Detailed summary tables and epidemiological commentary are available in the ES-PAUR report. Other topics covered within the AMR chapter include results from the Gonococcal Resistance to Antimicrobials Surveillance Programme (GRASP), AMR in tuberculosis, antifungal resistance, antiviral resistance, and details of participation in international AMR surveillance.

4. Discussion

Whilst a 10.8% increase in patient episodes of bacteraemia or fungaemia was observed between 2017 and 2021, the incidence rate change varied for different pathogens, particularly with the decrease in *E. coli* and *S. pneumoniae* BSI (74.3/100,000 population to 66.9 and 8.7 to 4.0, respectively) seen in 2020 and 2021. The decreased rates of BSI seen for *E. coli* and *S. pneumoniae* are likely due, at least in part, to the COVID-19 pandemic and associated public health interventions. This resulted in reduced contact between individuals and overall fewer interactions with the healthcare system, such as cancellation of elective surgery or access to GP consultations, although the underlying causes of reductions in BSI rates are likely to be complex and multifactorial. *E. coli* contributes substantially to the total BSI burden, and the marked reduction in BSI incidence may also be due to changes in healthcare interactions in vulnerable populations and antibiotic usage [5], therefore driving the 4.2% decrease in the burden of resistance between 2017 and 2021, although this was not significant. In contrast, other Gram-negative species causing BSI increased between 2017 and 2021, partly due to the more hospital-onset nature of *Klebsiella* spp. and *Pseudomonas aeruginosa* [9]. As we emerge from the COVID-19 pandemic, it will take time to assess the resulting impact on bacterial trends and the AMR burden, particularly in light of the decreasing overall numbers (but the increasing rate per 1000 occupied bed-days) of total blood cultures [8]. The burden of resistant infections remained relatively unchanged for Gram-positive infections overall. The diverging CFR, with higher CFR rates linked with increased resistance, will require further monitoring and investigation, as the true picture is more nuanced than resistance alone and will be affected, for example, by population demographics, comorbidity, time to effective treatment, and pathogenicity.

The detected regional differences in the AMR burden, and carbapenemase family prevalence and distribution, require local and regional knowledge, context, and strategies to understand and target healthcare interventions. Additionally, the effect of deprivation on CPO incidence and the effect of the AMR burden across ethnic groups have been described for the first time in this chapter. While the majority of resistant BSI were recorded in those with White ethnicity (80.8%), this percentage is lower than the national population (84.8%), and 'Asian, Asian British' accounts for 7.4% the population and only 6.1% of the resistant BSI reports; however, ethnic group population rates vary by region and rurality [10]. Understanding the impact of ethnicity, deprivation, and regional divergence, along with potential confounders, remains a crucial avenue of enquiry, and these investigations are currently underway using data linkage and form one of the future actions of this report.

Author Contributions: Conceptualization, R.G. and S.M.G.; methodology, R.G.; validation, R.G., K.L.H. (Katherine L. Henderson), H.H. and J.R.; formal analysis, H.F., K.F.B., H.H., R.G. and J.R.; investigation, H.H., K.L.H. (Katherine L. Henderson) and K.L.H. (Katie L. Hopkins); writing—original draft preparation, R.G.; writing—review and editing, K.L.H. (Katherine L. Henderson), S.M.G., M.M. and H.H.; visualization, R.G.; supervision, S.M.G., A.D. and K.L.H. (Katherine L. Henderson). All authors have read and agreed to the published version of the manuscript.

Funding: This research received no external funding.

Institutional Review Board Statement: Not applicable.

Informed Consent Statement: Patient consent was not sought under Section 251 of the National Health Service Act 2006.

Data Availability Statement: The data presented in this study are available in [5].

Acknowledgments: We would like to thank Daniele Meunier, Gauri Godbole, Suzy Sun, Elizabeth Johnson, Riina Rautemaa-Richardson, Daniel Bradshaw, Tamyo Mbisa, Samreen Ljaz, Esther Robinson, and Sharon Cox for their contributions and expertise during the compilation of the annual update on AMR in ESPAUR. In addition, the participation of the NHS laboratories in the routine laboratory surveillance of infections in England is essential for the greater understanding of AMR in England, and they should be thanked.

Conflicts of Interest: The authors declare no conflict of interest.

References

1. Murray, C.J.; Ikuta, K.S.; Sharara, F.; Swetschinski, L.; Robles Aguilar, G.; Gray, A.; Han, C.; Bisignano, C.; Rao, P.; Wool, E.; et al. Global Burden of Bacterial Antimicrobial Resistance in 2019: A Systematic Analysis. *Lancet* **2022**, *399*, 629–655. [CrossRef] [PubMed]
2. *Annual Report of the Chief Medical Officer, Volume Two, 2011, Infections and the Rise of Antimicrobial Resistance*; Department of Health and Social Care: London, UK, 2012.
3. *Tackling Antimicrobial Resistance 2019 to 2024: The UK's 5-Year National Action Plan*; Department of Health and Social Care: London, UK, 2019.
4. *Contained and Controlled: The UK's 20-Year Vision for Antimicrobial Resistance*; Department of Health and Social Care: London, UK, 2019.
5. Guy, R.; Higgins, H.; Rudman, J.; Fountain, H.; Henderson, K.L.; Bennet, K.; Hopkins, K.L.; Gerver, S.M.; Mirfenderesky, M. Chapter 2 Antimicrobial resistance (AMR). In *English Surveillance Programme for Antimicrobial Utilisation and Resistance (ESPAUR) Report 2021 to 22*; UK Health Security Agency: London, UK, 2022.
6. Cassini, A.; Hogberg, L.D.; Plachouras, D.; Quattrocchi, A.; Hoxha, A.; Simonsen, G.S.; Colomb-Cotinat, M.; Kretzschmar, M.E.; Devleesschauwer, B.; Cecchini, M.; et al. Attributable Deaths and Disability-Adjusted Life-Years Caused by Infections with Antibiotic-Resistant Bacteria in the EU and the European Economic Area in 2015: A Population-Level Modelling Analysis. *Lancet Infect. Dis.* **2019**, *19*, 56–66. [CrossRef] [PubMed]
7. Method for Assigning Ethnic Group in the COVID-19 Health Inequalities Monitoring for England (CHIME) Tool. Available online: https://www.gov.uk/government/statistics/covid-19-health-inequalities-monitoring-in-england-tool-chime/method-for-assigning-ethnic-group-in-the-covid-19-health-inequalities-monitoring-for-england-chime-tool (accessed on 6 August 2022).
8. Blood Culture Sets per 1,000 Bed-Days Performed by Reporting Acute Trust and Quarter. Available online: https://fingertips.phe.org.uk/profile/amr-local-indicators/data#page/4/gid/1938132910/pat/159/par/K02000001/ati/15/are/E92000001/iid/92331/age/1/sex/4/cat/-1/ctp/-1/yrr/1/cid/4/tbm/1 (accessed on 14 April 2022).
9. Sloot, R.; Nsonwu, O.; Chudasama, D.; Rooney, G.; Pearson, C.; Choi, H.; Mason, E.; Springer, A.; Gerver, S.; Brown, C.; et al. Rising Rates of Hospital-Onset Klebsiella Spp. and Pseudomonas Aeruginosa Bacteraemia in NHS Acute Trusts in England: A Review of National Surveillance Data, August 2020–February 2021. *J. Hosp. Infect.* **2022**, *119*, 175–181. [CrossRef] [PubMed]
10. Statistical Digest of Rural England. Available online: https://www.gov.uk/government/statistics/statistical-digest-of-rural-england (accessed on 20 February 2023).

Disclaimer/Publisher's Note: The statements, opinions and data contained in all publications are solely those of the individual author(s) and contributor(s) and not of MDPI and/or the editor(s). MDPI and/or the editor(s) disclaim responsibility for any injury to people or property resulting from any ideas, methods, instructions or products referred to in the content.

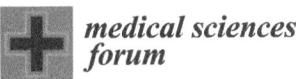

Abstract

Antimicrobial Consumption in England, 2017 to 2021 †

Sabine Bou-Antoun [1,*], Angela Falola [1], Holly Fountain [1], Hanna Squire [1], Colin S. Brown [1], Susan Hopkins [1], Sarah M. Gerver [1] and Alicia Demirjian [1,2,3]

1. United Kingdom Health Security Agency (UKHSA), London NW9 5EQ, UK
2. Department of Paediatric Infectious Diseases & Immunology, Evelina London Children's Hospital, London SE1 7EH, UK
3. Faculty of Life Sciences & Medicine, King's College London, London WC2R 2LS, UK
* Correspondence: sabine.bou-antoun@ukhsa.gov.uk
† Presented at the ESPAUR 2021/22 Webinar, Antibiotic Guardian, 23 November 2022. Available online: https://antibioticguardian.com/Meetings/espaur-2021-22-webinar/.

Abstract: The UK's 5-year National Action Plan for Antimicrobial Resistance has an ambition to reduce total antimicrobial consumption, a key driver of antimicrobial resistance, in humans by 15% by 2024, highlighting the need for active surveillance to inform on progression. The English Surveillance Programme for Antimicrobial Utilisation and Resistance (ESPAUR) report, Chapter 3, commentates on key national antimicrobial consumption trends, across primary and secondary care in England, between 2017 to 2021. These findings were presented at the ESPAUR Report webinar on 23 November 2022.

Keywords: antimicrobial consumption; antibiotic; antifungal; England

1. Introduction

Antimicrobial resistance (AMR) is a recognised global public health threat. Concerns around growing antimicrobial resistance and a dwindling antimicrobial pipeline have placed a focus on AMR at the United Nations General Assembly, and at the G7 and G20 summits [1]. The UK Government has committed to reducing inappropriate antimicrobial consumption, a key driver of resistance, through the National Action Plan; with an ambition to reduce total antimicrobial consumption in humans by 15% by 2024 [2]. In the last seven years, the work of the English Surveillance Programme for Antimicrobial Utilisation and Resistance (ESPAUR), collaborators and stakeholders have supported the ambitions and seen a reduction in total antibiotic use by almost 20%. The ESPAUR report, Chapter 3, commentates on the continued monitoring of trends in antimicrobial usage, over time (including during the COVID-19 pandemic) and across different prescribing settings [3,4].

2. Methods

2.1. Data and Data Sources

Data on the use of antimicrobials (antibiotics, antifungals and antimalarials) were obtained from two main data sources: ePACT2 from the NHS Business Services Authority for antibiotics prescribed in primary care (including NHS dental surgeries), and IQVIA for secondary care. The database held by IQVIA contains data from 99% of NHS hospital pharmacy systems for drugs dispensed to individual patients and wards. Data from all NHS acute Trusts were included.

The covered prescribing settings were general practice (GP), other community settings such as out-of-hours services and walk-in centres, dental practice, and hospital inpatient and outpatient services (ESPAUR Chapter 3 Annexe for further details) [4].

Mid-year populations (inhabitants) were extracted from the Office for National Statistics (ONS). Hospital admission data for each year were extracted from Hospital Episode Statistics (HES) from NHS Digital.

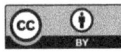

2.2. Data Processing and Statistical Analyses

Depending on the healthcare setting assessed, antimicrobial consumption was measured as items or Defined Daily Doses (DDDs). Rates were calculated as items per 1000 inhabitants per day, or DDDs per 1000 inhabitants per day (DID), or DDDs per 1000 hospital admissions. DDDs were calculated using the Anatomical Therapeutic Chemical/Daily Defined Dose (ATC/DDD) index 2019 managed by the World Health Organisation (WHO). Antibiotic data covered all antibiotics in the ATC group 'J01' ('Antibiotics for systemic use') and additional oral agents used to treat *Clostridium difficile* infections: fidamoxicin (A07AA12), metronidazole (P01AB01), tinidazole (P01AB02) and vancomycin (A07AA09).

Antifungal data covered all antifungals in the ATC group 'J02' ('Antimycotics for systemic use'), and one additional systemic antifungal, terbinafine (D01BA02) [4].

National trends in the consumption of antimicrobials were assessed using linear regression, where the dependent variable was antimicrobial consumption as DID and the explanatory variable was year. STATA version 17 (STATA Corp, College Station, TX, USA) was used to perform the data management and analyses.

3. Results

3.1. Total Antibiotic Consumption

In England, total antibiotic consumption (DDDs per 1000 inhabitants per day [DID]) had been decreasing between 2017 and 2019 (−4.3%, from 18.80 to 17.99 DID), with a sharp and substantial decline seen coinciding with the COVID-19 pandemic (−10.9% between 2019 and 2020 alone), followed by a further 0.5% decline between 2020 to 2021 (from 16.02 to 15.95 DID). This reduction was consistent across all UKHSA centres, regardless of persistent regional variations seen (Figures 1 and 2a). In 2021, the three most commonly prescribed antibiotic groups continued to be penicillins (36.7%), tetracyclines (27.1%) and "macrolides, lincosamides and streptogramins" (13.8%) [4]. Declines seen across all antibiotic groups (apart from oral metronidazole) in 2020 have continued in most antibiotic groups between 2020 and 2021, apart from significant increases noted for penicillins (excluding BLIs), carbapenems, anti-Clostridioides difficile agents, and 'other antibacterials' [4]. Consumption for these classes remained lower than 2019 levels.

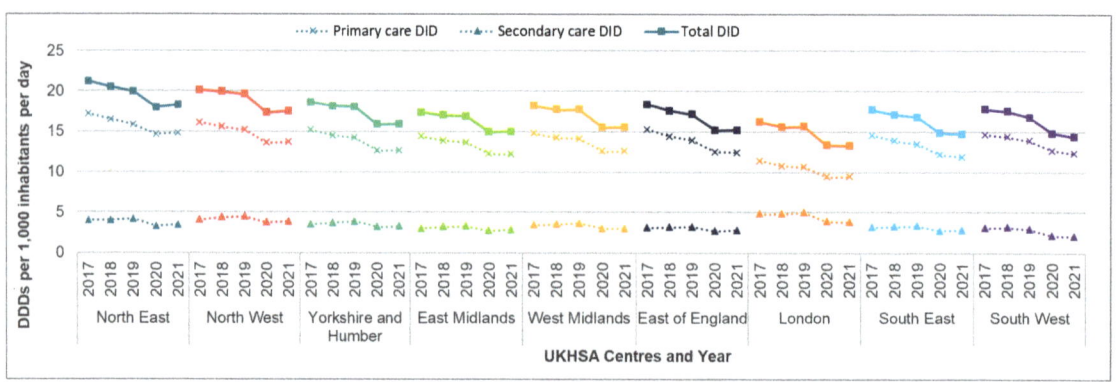

Figure 1. Total, primary and secondary care antibiotic consumption in UKHSA centres, 2017 to 2021 (Excludes dental practice data).

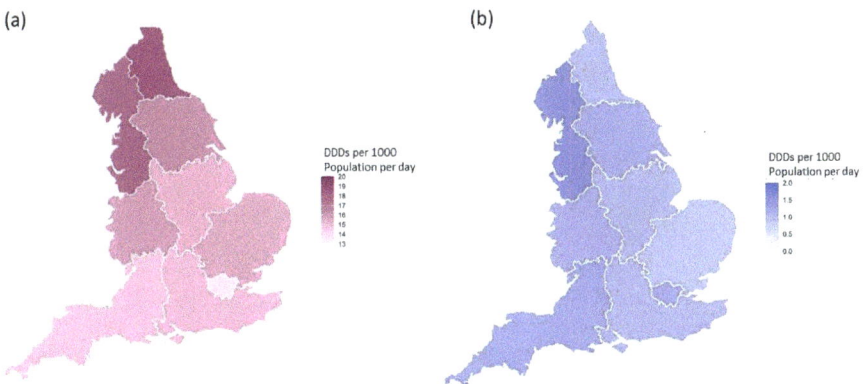

Figure 2. Total consumption of systemic (**a**) antibiotics and (**b**) antifungals across UKHSA centres in England, 2021.

3.1.1. Primary Care Antibiotic Consumption

Across the five years, total and broad-spectrum prescribing rates within primary care continued to decline. Prescribing increases were noted in general practice (0.5%, from 1.245 to 1.251 items per 1000 inhabitants per day) and other community setting prescribing (18%, from 0.081 to 0.096 items per 1000 inhabitants per day) between 2020 and 2021, however, rates remained lower than 2019 [4]. Declines in primary care broad-spectrum antibiotic prescribing rates continued, with a large decrease of 19.8% observed between 2019 and 2020 (0.59 to 0.48 items per 1000 inhabitants per day) and a subsequent increase of 5.6% in 2021 (to 0.50 items per 1000 inhabitants per day), this remaining below 2019 levels [4]. In 2021, the three most predominantly prescribed antibiotic groups in general practices were, as in previous years, penicillins (45.2%), tetracyclines (15.7%), and other antibacterials (15.5%) [4].

From 2017 to 2020 there had been a general decrease in gerenal practice items per 1000 inhabitants per day across all age groups. In 2021, compared with 2020, there were increases amongst the 0–4, 5–14 and 15–64 years age categories (greatest increase amongst 0–4 years: +51.8%, from 0.94 to 1.42 items per 1000 inhabitants per day). This followed a large reduction in prescribing for children aged 0–4 years in 2020 (−39.9%), and is now more in line with 2019 rates. The usage rates in the elderly age groups (65+ years) continued to decrease [4].

Consumption in NHS dental practices, following an unusual 17.6% increase (particulalry in amoxicillin and metronidazole) between 2019 and 2020 (0.13 to 0.15 items per 1000 inhabitants per day), decreased (−7.1%, to 0.14 items per 1000 inhabitants per day in 2021), albietly this was still higher than pre-pandemic levels [4].

3.1.2. Secondary Care Antibiotic Consumption

In 2021, the antibiotic prescribing rate (4372 DDDs per 1000 admissions) in secondary care had decreased by 5.2% compared to 2017, and by 10.4% compared to 2020. There were similar decreases in prescribing rates from 2017 to 2021 across all acute Trust types. In 2020, there were large increases in prescribing rate (DDDs per 1000 admissions) in acute Trusts, likely due to the COVID-19 pandemic, changes in hospital admissions and case-mix of patients (this increased rate masks what was a decline in DDDs during this period and a greater decline in hospital admissions, the denominator), which have since decreased in 2021. Reductions were particularly pronounced among acute large (−16.5% from 2020 to 2021) and acute specialist (−13.7%) Trusts [4].

The antibiotic classes with the highest use in secondary care (comprising approximately one-fifth of prescribing of secondary care antibiotics assessed) in 2021 were 'penicillins (beta-lactam inhibitor combinations only)' and 'penicillins (excluding beta-lactam inhibitor combinations)' [4]. All antibiotic groups decreased in DDDs per 1000 admissions from 2020 to 2021, except for anti-Clostridioides difficile agents, which increased by 9.2% (5.4 to 5.9 DDDs per 1000 admissions) [4].

According to WHO's Access, Watch and Reserve (AWaRe) categories, adapted to fit England's prescribing environment [5], 'Access' antibiotics were prescribed the most in 2021 (53.1% out of the total DDDs per 1000 admissions), followed by 'Watch' (45.3%) and 'Reserve' (3.1%). These percentages are similar to previous years [4].

3.2. Antifungal Consumption

Total antifungal consumption (primary and secondary care) increased by 7.1% to 1.03 DID from 2020 to 2021, this was still lower than in 2017 by 22.9%. Systemic antifungal use is mostly driven by use in primary care, with 87% of prescribing taking place in this setting in 2021 (0.9 DID). There was a 25.4% decrease in primary care antifungal use from the rate in 2017, but a 6.9% increase from 2020. In secondary care the rate of prescribing was 191 DDDs per 1000 admissions in 2021, representing a 7.1% increase from 2017, but a 4.5% decrease from the rate in 2020 [4].

In 2021, the North West had the highest total antifungal prescribing rate (1.37 DID), whilst the East of England had the lowest (0.81 DID) (Figure 2b). Terbinafine had the highest rate of antifungal prescribing in primary care (2021: 0.67 DID), whilst fluconazole was the highest in secondary care (2021: 67 DDDs per 1000 admissions per day).

4. Discussion

Continued declines in total antibiotic consumption were observed, with a sharp decline between 2019 and 2020 (10.9%), and a slighter decrease of 0.5% between 2020 and 2021. In addition to improvements in antimicrobial stewardship and progress towards the NAP targets, this decreasing trend highlights the impact that the COVID-19 pandemic has had on antimicrobial consumption in England. The most recent 2021 data suggest that this may not be a sustained change [4]. The largest reductions in antibiotic prescribing have consistently been within the GP setting, which is also the setting in which the highest level of antibiotic consumption occurs [4]. The large reductions in prescribing in 2020 in the 0–4 year old patients are likely related to reduced respiratory antibiotic prescribing in the young [6] and reduced general practice consultations [7] related to national COVID-19 prevention measures. Following this steep reduction, in 2021, there were increases amongst the younger age groups (greatest amongst 0–4 years old; +51.7%) and is more in line with 2019 rates [4]. Despite improved infection prevention measures by health care professionals and general population alike and changes in service delivery (fewer face-to-face consultations in primary care and less hospital admissions, particularly during the first year of the COVID-19 pandemic), there were other factors which would have altered prescribing needs and behaviours, such as; social restrictions encouraged through national and regional 'lock-down' measures (increased household spread of infections), wearing of masks impacting circulation of pathogens, and changes in the case mix of patients consulting in primary care (reduction in appointments for the very young) as well as those admitted into hospital (with delayed and cancelled elective procedures and increases in more acutely ill patients and admissions to intensive care and high dependency units). With services beginning to resume, consumption trends are somewhat changing to reflect this in 2021 [4].

COVID-19 restrictions and reduced access to dentistry in England had the opposing impact on antibiotic prescribing trends to other primary care settings, with published literature also demonstrating unprecedented increases in this setting between 2019 and 2020, which are now beginning to reduce [8].

Across settings, significant increases were noted for penicillins (excluding BLIs), carbapenems, anti-*Clostridioides difficile* agents, and 'other antibacterials' between 2020 and 2021 [4]. During this same period, secondary care use reduced across all antibiotic groups, except for anti-*Clostridioides difficile*. The increase in carbapenems is likely related to their inclusion within national guidelines [4,9,10]. Increased use in anti-*Clostridioides difficile* agents may be related to noted increases in hospital-onset *Clostridioides difficile* infections reported [4,11].

Total antifungal consumption did not demonstrate a decrease between 2020 and 2021 as was seen with antibiotic use. While it is not possible to further describe these trends without indication data, the literature reports antifungal agents have been administered as prophylaxis or combination therapy among COVID-19 patients [12]. This may be related to the increasing prevalence of invasive fungal infections (usually acquired by immunocompromised patients in hospitals and in the ICU settings) [4].

5. Conclusions

The UKHSA continues to work alongside key stakeholders to bring together relevant information to inform on trends and the impact of various factors on antimicrobial prescribing, and progress towards the NAP. Improvements and reductions in prescribing have been made, although we are seeing increases in consumption returning towards pre-pandemic levels since healthcare services have resumed activities. Continued stewardship and surveillance are therefore needed for sustained progress in reducing antimicrobial consumption as systems continue to recover from the COVID-19 pandemic.

Author Contributions: Conceptualization, S.B.-A.; methodology, A.F., H.F. and S.B.-A.; validation, H.S. and S.B.-A.; formal analysis: A.F., H.F., H.S. and S.B.-A.; investigation, S.B.-A., A.F., H.F., S.M.G.; writing—original draft preparation, S.B.-A., A.F. and H.F.; writing—review and editing, S.B.-A., A.D., S.M.G., S.H., C.S.B.; supervision, S.B.-A. and A.D. All authors have read and agreed to the published version of the manuscript.

Funding: This research received no external funding.

Data Availability Statement: The data presented in this study are available in [Bou-Antoun, S.; Falola, A.; Fountain, H.; Squire, H.; Budd, E.; Brown, C.S.; Hopkins, S.; Gerver, S.M. The English Surveillance Programme for Antimicrobial Utilisation and Resistance (ESPAUR) report 2020 to 2021, Chapter 5 Antimicrobial Consumption, London, 2021.] and the reports' supplementary material.

Acknowledgments: The authors would like to acknowledge the ESPAUR Oversight Group members.

Conflicts of Interest: The authors declare no conflict of interest.

References

1. Mendelson, M.; Sharland, M.; Mpundu, M. Antibiotic resistance: Calling time on the 'silent pandemic'. *JAC Antimicrob Resist* **2022**, *4*, dlac016. [CrossRef] [PubMed]
2. *UK 5-Year Action Plan for Antimicrobial Resistance 2019 to 2024*; Department of Health and Social Care: London, UK, 2019.
3. Ashiru-Oredope, D.; Susan Hopkins on behalf of the English Surveillance Programme for Antimicrobial Utilization and Resistance Oversight Group; Kessel, A.; Hopkins, S.; Ashiru-Oredope, D.; Brown, B.; Brown, N.; Carter, S.; Charlett, A.; Cichowka, A.; et al. Antimicrobial stewardship: English surveillance programme for antimicrobial utilization and resistance (ESPAUR). *J. Antimicrob. Chemother.* **2013**, *68*, 2421–2423. [PubMed]
4. Bou-Antoun, S.; Falola, A.; Fountain, H.; Squire, H.; Brown, C.S.; Hopkins, S.; Gerver, S.M.; Demirjian, A. *The English Surveillance Programme for Antimicrobial Utilisation and Resistance (ESPAUR) Report 2021 to 2022, Chapter 3 Antimicrobial Consumption*; UK Health Security Agency: London, UK, 2022.
5. Budd, E.; Cramp, E.; Sharland, M.; Hand, K.; Howard, P.; Wilson, P.; Wilcox, M.; Muller-Pebody, B.; Hopkins, S. Adaptation of the WHO Essential Medicines List for national antibiotic stewardship policy in England: Being AWaRe. *JAC* **2019**, *74*, 3384–3389. [CrossRef] [PubMed]
6. Andrews, A.; Bou-Antoun, S.; Guy, R.; Brown, C.S.; Hopkins, S.; Gerver, S. Respiratory antibacterial prescribing in primary care and the COVID-19 pandemic in England, winter season 2020–21. *JAC* **2022**, *77*, 799–802. [CrossRef] [PubMed]
7. Bou-Antoun, S.; Falola, A.; Fountain, H.; Squire, H.; Budd, E.; Brown, C.S.; Hopkins, S.; Gerver, S.M. *The English Surveillance Programme for Antimicrobial Utilisation and Resistance (ESPAUR) report 2020 to 2021, Chapter 5 Antimicrobial Consumption*; UK Health Security Agency: London, UK, 2021.
8. Shah, S.; Wordley, V.; Thompson, W. How did COVID-19 impact on dental antibiotic prescribing across England? *Br. Dent. J.* **2020**, *229*, 601–604, Erratum in: *Br. Dent. J.* **2022**, *232*, 303–306. [CrossRef] [PubMed]
9. The National Institute for Health and Care Excellence (NICE). *Pneumonia (Hospital-Acquired): Antimicrobial Prescribing NICE guideline*; NG139; UK Health Security Agency: London, UK, 2019.

10. *COVID-19 Rapid Guideline: Antibiotics for Pneumonia in Adults in Hospital*; NG173; UK Health Security Agency: London, UK, 2020.
11. UKHSA National Statistics: Annual Epidemiological Commentary: Gram-Negative, MRSA, MSSA Bacteraemia and C. Difficile Infections, up to and including Financial Year 2021 to 2022. Available online: https://www.gov.uk/search/research-and-statistics (accessed on 31 December 2022).
12. Hatzl, S.; Reisinger, A.C.; Posch, F.; Prattes, J.; Stradner, M.; Pilz, S.; Eller, P.; Schoerghuber, M.; Toller, W.; Gorkiewicz, G.; et al. Antifungal prophylaxis for prevention of COVID-19-associated pulmonary aspergillosis in critically ill patients: An observational study. *Crit. Care* **2021**, *25*, 335. [CrossRef] [PubMed]

Disclaimer/Publisher's Note: The statements, opinions and data contained in all publications are solely those of the individual author(s) and contributor(s) and not of MDPI and/or the editor(s). MDPI and/or the editor(s) disclaim responsibility for any injury to people or property resulting from any ideas, methods, instructions or products referred to in the content.

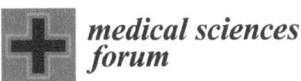

Proceeding Paper

ESPAUR Report 2021 to 2022 Chapter 5: NHS England Improvement and Assurance Schemes [†]

Kieran Hand [1,*], Diane Ashiru-Oredope [2], Elizabeth Beech [1], Sabine Bou-Antoun [2], Gillian Damant [1], Naomi Fleming [1], Catherine Hayes [2], Philip Howard [1], Conor Jamieson [1], Monsey McLeod [1], Sejal Parekh [3], Preety Ramdut [1], Hanna Squire [2], Laura Whitney [1] and Jeff Featherstone [4,*]

[1] Antimicrobial Prescribing and Medicines Optimisation (APMO) Workstream, AMR Programme, NHS England, London SE1 8UG, UK
[2] HCAI, Fungal, AMR, AMU & Sepsis Division, UK Health Security Agency, London SW1P 3HX, UK
[3] Community Services and Strategy Directorate, Primary Care, NHS England, London SE1 8UG, UK
[4] AMR Programme, NHS England, Leeds LS2 7UE, UK
* Correspondence: kieran.hand@nhs.net (K.H.); jefffeatherstone@nhs.net (J.F.)
[†] Presented at the ESPAUR 2021/22 Webinar, Antibiotic Guardian, 23 November 2022; Available online: https://antibioticguardian.com/Meetings/espaur-2021-22-webinar/.

Abstract: NHS England designs and administers improvement and assurance schemes that include elements to incentivize prudent use of antimicrobials, optimise patient outcomes, minimise avoidable exposure to antimicrobials, and reduce selection pressure for antimicrobial resistance (AMR). These schemes include the NHS System Oversight Framework, the Pharmacy Quality Scheme for community pharmacies, the NHS Standard Contract, and the Commissioning for Quality and Innovation (CQUIN) framework. This report describes the schemes implemented from 2021 to 2022, and it reports the scheme performance of NHS commissioners and healthcare provider organisations. A summary of improvement and assurance schemes from 2022 to 2023 is also provided.

Keywords: antimicrobial stewardship; antimicrobial resistance; policy; prescribing; medicines optimisation; improvement; assurance

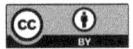

1. Introduction

This report summarises improvement and assurance schemes relevant to antimicrobial use that are designed and administered by NHS England through contractual frameworks with healthcare commissioners and providers and reported in the annual report of the English Surveillance Programme for Antimicrobial Use and Resistance (ESPAUR) [1]. The schemes aim to incentivize the prudent use of antimicrobials to optimise patient outcomes, minimise avoidable exposure to antimicrobials, and reduce selection pressure for antimicrobial resistance (AMR).

2. Primary Care—Reducing Avoidable Antibiotic Prescribing

2.1. The NHS System Oversight Framework

The NHS System Oversight Framework provides clarity to integrated care systems, acute hospital trusts and commissioners on how NHS England will monitor performance, sets expectations on working together to maintain and improve the quality of care, and describes how identified support needs will be addressed to improve standards and how outcomes will be coordinated and delivered [2]. Integrated care systems (ICSs) are partnerships of organisations that come together to plan and deliver joined-up health and care services and to improve the lives of people who live and work in their area.

2.2. The NHS System Oversight Framework Metrics and Targets for 2021–2022

The NHS System Oversight Framework from 2021 to 2022 includes two AMR-related metrics, both applicable to primary care. Clinical Commissioning Groups—*Antimicrobial resistance: appropriate prescribing of antibiotics and broad-spectrum antibiotics in primary care*. Clinical commissioning groups (CCGs) were created in England following the Health and Social Care Act in 2012 and replaced primary care trusts on 1 April 2013. They were clinically-led statutory NHS bodies responsible for the planning and commissioning of health care services for their local area. As of 1 April 2021, following a series of mergers, there were 106 CCGs in England. However, they were dissolved in July 2022, and their duties were taken on by the new integrated care systems (ICSs). The metrics and associated targets are set out in Table 1. The target for total prescribing of antibiotics is aligned with the UK AMR National Action Plan's (2019–2024) ambition to reduce community antibiotic prescribing by 25% from a 2013 baseline by 2024 [3].

Table 1. NHS System Oversight metrics and targets for antibiotic prescribing.

Code	AMR Metric Description	Target [1]
SO44a	Antimicrobial resistance: total prescribing of antibiotics in primary care. The number of antibiotic (antibacterial) items prescribed in primary care, divided by the item-based Specific Therapeutic Group Age-Sex Related Prescribing Unit (STAR-PU) per annum.	At or less than 0.871 items per STAR-PU
SO44b	Antimicrobial resistance: proportion of broad-spectrum antibiotic prescribing in primary care. The number of broad-spectrum antibiotic (antibacterial) items from co-amoxiclav, cephalosporin class, and fluoroquinolone class drugs as a percentage of the total number of antibacterial items prescribed in primary care.	At or less than 10%

[1] Target achievement date: 31 March 2024.

2.3. Performance against the NHS System Oversight Framework for 2021–2022

Human exposure to antibiotics in primary care is expressed as the number of prescription items (numerator) per registered patient (denominator) adjusted for population age and sex demographics using the Specific Therapeutic Group Age-Sex Related Prescribing Unit (STAR-PU) system. [4] For the 12 months to 31 March 2022, the number of ICSs meeting the target for total prescribing of antibiotics at or less than 0.871 items per STAR-PU was 21/42 (50%) and the number of ICSs meeting the target for broad-spectrum antibiotic prescribing at or less than 10% was 35/42 (83%). The number of ICSs meeting both targets was 17/42 (40%).

For the 12 months to 31 March 2022, the number of CCGs meeting the target for total prescribing of antibiotics at or less than 0.871 items per STAR-PU was 36/106 (34%), and the number of CCGs meeting the target for broad-spectrum antibiotic prescribing less than 10% was 89/106 (84%). The number of CCGs meeting both targets was 29/106 (27%).

3. Community Pharmacy—The NHS Pharmacy Quality Scheme

3.1. The Pharmacy Quality Scheme

The Pharmacy Quality Scheme (PQS) forms part of the Community Pharmacy Contractual Framework (CPCF) for England. It supports the delivery of the NHS Long Term Plan and rewards community pharmacy contractors that deliver quality criteria in three quality dimensions: clinical effectiveness, patient safety, and patient experience [5].

3.2. The Pharmacy Quality Scheme Metrics and Targets for 2021–2022

The Antimicrobial Stewardship (AMS) criterion of the 2021–2022 Pharmacy Quality Scheme included a rollout of the Treat Antibiotics Responsibly, Guidance, Education, and Tools (TARGET) Antibiotic Checklist to community pharmacies in England [6]. Pharmacy teams were required to submit evidence that they had reviewed their current AMS practise using the TARGET Antibiotic Checklist, to be carried out over four weeks with a minimum of 25 patients, or up to eight weeks if the minimum number of patients was not achieved within four weeks. 74% of community pharmacies in England submitted audit data, and 213,105 checklists were completed with patients.

3.3. Performance agains the Pharmacy Quality Scheme for 2021–2022

The PQS ran from 1 September 2021 to 31 March 2022, and in that time, 8374 community pharmacies submitted evidence to the UKHSA portal from 213,105 antibiotic prescriptions assessed with the TARGET Antibiotic Checklist.

4. Secondary Care—Reducing Avoidable Antibiotic Prescribing in NHS Trust Providers of Acute Care

4.1. The NHS Standard Contract

The planned NHS Standard Contract from 2020 to 2021 was suspended in March 2020 in response to the COVID-19 pandemic.

4.2. The NHS Standard Contract Metrics and Targets for 2021–2022

An antibiotic consumption reduction target was reinstated within the NHS Standard Contract from 2021 to 2022 for all NHS Trusts providing acute care, with a target to reduce antibiotic consumption by 2% from each Trust's 2018 calendar year baseline value [7].

4.3. Performance against the NHS Standard Contract for 2021–2022

An overview of changes to antibiotic consumption targets, scope, and performance against targets is provided in Table 2. From 2021 to 2022, 69/138 (50%) of participating NHS Trusts met the target to reduce total antibiotic consumption by 2% from 2018, and antibiotic consumption across all participating Trusts at financial year end was 4465 DDD per 1000 admissions.

Table 2. Summary of changes to NHS Standard Contract antibiotic consumption targets and achievement from 2019 to 2022.

Contract Year	Target Reduction in Antibiotic Consumption from Calendar Year 2018 Baseline	Number of Trusts that Met Requirement	Antibiotic Consumption Value at Year End
2019–2020	1% reduction in total DDD [1] per 1000 admissions (cf. 2018)	43/145 (30%)	4612 DDD per 1000 admissions
2020–2021	Suspended due to COVID-19 pandemic	N/A	N/A
2021–2022	2% reduction in total DDD per 1000 admissions (cf. 2018)	69/138 (50%)	4465 DDD per 1000 admissions
2022–2023	4.5% reduction in DDD per 1000 admissions for antibiotics from the WHO "Watch" and "Reserve" categories (cf. 2018)	Current	Current

[1] World Health Organisation Defined Daily Doses.

5. Secondary Care—Commissioning for Quality and Innovation (CQUIN)

The Commissioning for Quality and Innovation (CQUIN) framework supports improvements in the quality of services and the creation of new, improved patterns of care. The CQUIN framework was suspended in March 2020 in response to the COVID-19 pandemic.

6. NHS England Plans from 2022 to 2023

6.1. FutureNHS AMR Programme Workspace

The NHS England AMR Programme Workspace was relaunched on the FutureNHS web-based platform in March 2022 to support local, regional, and national stakeholders to access guidance, resources (including frequently asked questions), and performance data for national improvement and assurance schemes. Access to FutureNHS requires registration but is open to NHS staff with an nhs.net e-mail address [8]. Visits to the workspace by registered members have risen steadily since launch, peaking at 305 per month in August 2022.

6.2. NHS Oversight Framework from 2022 to 2023

The NHS Oversight Framework was relaunched for 2022–23, replacing the NHS System Oversight Framework for 2021–22. The NHS Oversight Framework reflects the significant changes enabled by the Health and Care Act 2022, including the formal establishment of Integrated Care Boards and the merging of NHS Improvement (comprising of Monitor and the NHS Trust Development Authority) into NHS England. The AMR metrics and targets for antibiotic prescribing set out in Table 1 (above) have been retained for the NHS Oversight Framework 2022–23 [9].

6.3. NHS Standard Contrct from 2022 to 2023

The scope of the antibiotic requirement in the NHS Standard Contract from 2022 to 2023 has been narrowed to antibiotics in the World Health Organisation (WHO) "Watch" and "Reserve" categories adapted for use in England [10,11]. This change brings the performance measure into alignment with the ambition set out in the UK AMR National Action Plan for 2019–2024 [3].

6.4. NHS Commissioning for Quality and Innovation (CQUIN) Framework from 2022 to 2023

The NHS England AMR Programme is responsible for two CQUIN indicators from 2022 to 2023—CCG2: Appropriate antibiotic prescribing for UTI in adults aged 16+; and CCG3: Recording of NEWS2 score, escalation time, and response time for unplanned critical care admissions [12].

Two additional CQUIN indicators from 2022 to 2023 are relevant to infection and antibiotic prescribing—CCG5: Treatment of community acquired pneumonia in line with the British Thoracic Society (BTS) care bundle; and CCG14: Assessment, diagnosis, and treatment of lower leg wounds.

Author Contributions: Conceptualization, K.H., J.F. and D.A.-O.; methodology, K.H., E.B. and D.A.-O.; formal analysis, S.B.-A., C.H., H.S., M.M. and S.P.; writing—original draft preparation, K.H., E.B., G.D., N.F., P.H., C.J., M.M., S.P., P.R. and L.W.; writing—review and editing, K.H. and J.F. All authors have read and agreed to the published version of the manuscript.

Funding: This research received no external funding.

Institutional Review Board Statement: Not applicable.

Informed Consent Statement: Not applicable.

Data Availability Statement: Supporting data can be found in the ESPAUR Report 2021 to 2022 and references below. Registration is required to access FutureNHS.

Acknowledgments: The support of NHS England National Clinical Directors—Mark Wilcox and Matt Inada-Kim—and of colleagues from the other workstreams of the NHS England AMR Programme and Primary Care Pharmacy team is gratefully acknowledged. The support of colleagues from the UK Health Security Agency AMR Division and from NHS Business Services Authority for data collection, analysis, and reporting is also gratefully acknowledged.

Conflicts of Interest: The authors declare no conflict of interest.

References

1. UK Health Security Agency. English Surveillance Programme for Antimicrobial Utilisation and Resistance (ESPAUR) Report 2021 to 2022. UK Health Security Agency: London, November 2022. Available online: https://www.gov.uk/government/publications/english-surveillance-programme-antimicrobial-utilisation-and-resistance-espaur-report (accessed on 27 March 2023).
2. NHS System Oversight Framework 2021/22. Available online: https://www.england.nhs.uk/publication/system-oversight-framework-2021-22/ (accessed on 27 March 2023).
3. *UK 5-Year Action Plan for Antimicrobial Resistance 2019 to 2024*; Department of Health and Social Care: London, UK, 2019.
4. Lloyd, D.C.; Harris, C.M.; Roberts, D.J. Specific therapeutic group age-sex related prescribing units (STAR-PUs): Weightings for analysing general practices' prescribing in England. *BMJ* **1995**, *311*, 991–994. [CrossRef] [PubMed]
5. Pharmacy Quality Scheme. Available online: https://www.england.nhs.uk/primary-care/pharmacy/pharmacy-quality-payments-scheme/ (accessed on 27 March 2023).
6. TARGET Antibiotic Checklist. Version 2. Available online: https://elearning.rcgp.org.uk/pluginfile.php/172227/mod_book/chapter/447/antibiotic-checklist-v2.pdf (accessed on 27 March 2023).
7. 2021/22 NHS Standard Contract. Available online: https://www.england.nhs.uk/nhs-standard-contract/previous-nhs-standard-contracts/21-22/ (accessed on 27 March 2023).
8. FutureNHS Website. Available online: https://future.nhs.uk/ (accessed on 27 March 2023).
9. NHS Oversight Framework 2022/23. Available online: https://www.england.nhs.uk/nhs-oversight-framework/ (accessed on 27 March 2023).
10. 2022/23 NHS Standard Contract. Available online: https://www.england.nhs.uk/nhs-standard-contract/ (accessed on 27 March 2023).
11. Budd, E.; Cramp, E.; Sharland, M.; Hand, K.; Howard, P.; Wilson, P.; Wilcox, M.; Muller-Pebody, B.; Hopkins, S. Adaptation of the WHO Essential Medicines List for national antibiotic stewardship policy in England: Being AWaRe. *J. Antimicrob. Chemother.* **2019**, *74*, 3384–3389. [CrossRef] [PubMed]
12. 2022/23 CQUIN. Available online: https://www.england.nhs.uk/nhs-standard-contract/cquin/2022-23-cquin/ (accessed on 27 March 2023).

Disclaimer/Publisher's Note: The statements, opinions and data contained in all publications are solely those of the individual author(s) and contributor(s) and not of MDPI and/or the editor(s). MDPI and/or the editor(s) disclaim responsibility for any injury to people or property resulting from any ideas, methods, instructions or products referred to in the content.

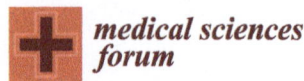

Proceeding Paper

National Antimicrobial Stewardship Activities in Primary and Secondary Care in England 2021–2022 (ESPAUR Report) †

Ella Casale [1], Catherine V. Hayes [1], Donna Lecky [1], Luke O'Neil [1], Eirwen Sides [1], Emily Cooper [1], Fionna Pursey [1], Sejal Parekh [2], Eleanor J. Harvey [1] and Diane Ashiru-Oredope [1,*]

1. HCAI, Fungal, AMR, AMU and Sepsis Division, UK Health Security Agency, London SW1P 3JR, UK
2. Primary Care, Community Services and Strategy Directorate, NHS England, London SE1 8UG, UK
* Correspondence: diane.ashiru-oredope@ukhsa.gov.uk
† Presented at the ESPAUR 2021/22 Webinar, Antibiotic Guardian, 23 November 2022; Available online: https://antibioticguardian.com/Meetings/espaur-2021-22-webinar/.

Abstract: A summary of key national primary and secondary care antimicrobial stewardship interventions led by the UK Health Security Agency (UKHSA) are highlighted. This includes development and implementation of TARGET Antibiotics Toolkit resources in community pharmacy and General Practice and the development of a national intravenous-to-oral switch (IVOS) criteria for use in secondary care.

Keywords: TARGET Antibiotic Checklist; AMS; community pharmacist; repeat antibiotics; antimicrobial

Citation: Casale, E.; Hayes, C.V.; Lecky, D.; O'Neil, L.; Sides, E.; Cooper, E.; Pursey, F.; Parekh, S.; Harvey, E.J.; Ashiru-Oredope, D. National Antimicrobial Stewardship Activities in Primary and Secondary Care in England 2021–2022 (ESPAUR Report). *Med. Sci. Forum* **2023**, *15*, 14. https://doi.org/10.3390/msf2022015014

Academic Editor: David Enoch

Published: 28 March 2023

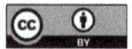

Copyright: © 2023 by the authors. Licensee MDPI, Basel, Switzerland. This article is an open access article distributed under the terms and conditions of the Creative Commons Attribution (CC BY) license (https://creativecommons.org/licenses/by/4.0/).

1. Introduction

Tackling antimicrobial resistance (AMR) requires action on multiple fronts to optimise antimicrobial use and reduce the emergence and transmission of resistance. An important element of this approach is the implementation of antimicrobial stewardship (AMS) interventions. AMS enables healthcare workers to choose the most appropriate drug, dosage and duration of treatment whilst limiting the microbe's ability to develop or acquire resistance. Optimising prescribing in this way is a key focus of the UK's 5-year National Action Plan on tackling AMR, which includes a target to reduce UK antimicrobial use in humans by 15% by 2024 [1].

The annual English Surveillance Programme for Antimicrobial Utilisation and Resistance (ESPAUR) report, Chapter 4, commentates on National AMS activities in primary and secondary care [2,3]. In this paper, we provide a summary of key national primary and secondary care antimicrobial stewardship interventions led by the UK Health Security Agency (UKHSA) and presented at the ESPAUR webinar on 23 November 2022 (https://antibioticguardian.com/Meetings/espaur-2021-22-webinar/, accessed on 23 March 2023).

2. Development and Implementation of TARGET Antibiotics Toolkit Resources for Primary Care and Community Pharmacy

2.1. Update of the TARGET Antibiotics Toolkit

The TARGET (Treat Antibiotics Responsibly, Guidance, Education, and Tools) antibiotics toolkit (Figure 1) is a suite of AMS resources to support primary care clinicians in championing and implementing AMS activities. The toolkit, designed and developed by UKHSA, is hosted on the Royal College of General Practitioners (RCGP) website [4]. The TARGET toolkit website underwent a major redesign in November 2021 to include new sections that provide evidence-based resources, supporting clinicians in discussing antibiotic use with patients. There were 167,827 views of the website from April 2021 to March 2022, with a peak in November coinciding with the website redesign and World Antimicrobial Awareness Week (WAAW). The 'leaflets to share with patients' [5] remained the most popular section of the TARGET Toolkit, and website-based HTML versions of the leaflets were introduced with the redesigned website. To help implement the HTML leaflets, UKHSA collaborated to develop templates with the company accuRx, which also produced software that allows GPs to communicate digitally with patients through text messages and emails.

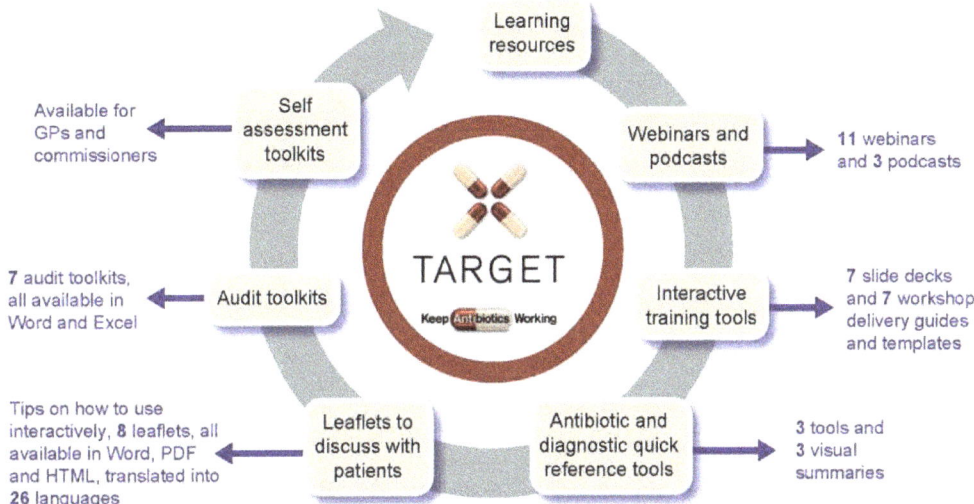

Figure 1. Resources included in the Treat Antibiotics Responsibly, Guidance, Education, and Tools (TARGET) Antibiotics Toolkit, available via Royal College of General Practitioners (www.rcgp.org.uk/targetantibiotics, accessed on 15 August 2022).

2.2. Implementation of the TARGET Antibiotic Checklist in Community Pharmacy

The TARGET Antibiotic Checklist [6], an AMS intervention for community pharmacy, was included as a criterion of the 2021–22 Pharmacy Quality Scheme (PQS). The PQS is an incentive scheme forming part of the community pharmacy contractual framework (CPCF) for all NHS community pharmacies in England [7]. Community pharmacy teams were required to use the checklist as part of their current antimicrobial practice for a period of four weeks with a minimum of 25 patients; or up to eight weeks if the minimum number of patients was not achieved within four weeks. Data were submitted from 8374 community pharmacies (74% of all pharmacies in England (11,133) at the time of the report) who used the TARGET Antibiotic Checklist with 213,105 antibiotic prescriptions dispensed to patients; 86% of the pharmacies entered data for at least the required 25 patients and 44% surpassed this. There was high engagement with this scheme, and the data provides an important understanding of AMS activities within community pharmacy.

2.3. Developing Tools for the Management of Long-Term and Repeated Antibiotic Use in General Practice

This work aimed to develop tools for healthcare professionals to review antibiotic use–specifically long-term and repeat antibiotics within general practice using a multi-step approach. In partnership with clinical pharmacists in primary care networks (PCNs) in England, the patient cohort that would benefit from the antimicrobial review was identified following the development of a search strategy to be conducted using GP electronic systems, EMIS and SystmOne. The aim was to identify patients with antimicrobials available on repeat prescription (long-term use) and/or issued over three courses in 6 months (repeat use). The search strategy also identified the top prescribed antimicrobials. This data informed which infections to focus on for initial management tools development. Data from OpenSAFELY was also requested and analysed to assess the most prescribed antimicrobials nationally.

The top antibiotic scripts (n = 225) issued for long-term and repeat use in a sample of PCNs included lymecycline (16%), oxytetracycline (12%), doxycycline (12%), amoxicillin (7%), and trimethoprim (7%). The most frequent infection indications were identified as acne (lymecycline/oxytetracycline) and respiratory tract infections, including those associated with chronic obstructive pulmonary disease (COPD) exacerbations (doxycycline/amoxicillin). Toolkits for acne and COPD exacerbations were developed, addressing the need for patient reviews and practice-based behaviour change to sustain AMS improvements.

3. Development of a National Intravenous-to-Oral Switch (IVOS) Criteria for Use in Secondary Care

Adult antibiotic IVOS policies from UK trusts were conveniently sampled for the collation of IVOS criteria. A literature search was undertaken in OVID Embase and Medline databases. Articles without IVOS criteria were excluded, as were those focusing on a specific antimicrobial or infection (for generalisable criteria).

Criteria available within trust guidelines, as well as from published literature, were entered into Excel spreadsheets. Those with the highest appearance informed a consensus of Delphi (Figure 2). Step 1) pilot/1st round questionnaire (24 respondents). Step 2) virtual meeting (15 participants) agreed to IVOS criteria. Step 3) 2nd round questionnaire (UK-wide cascade).

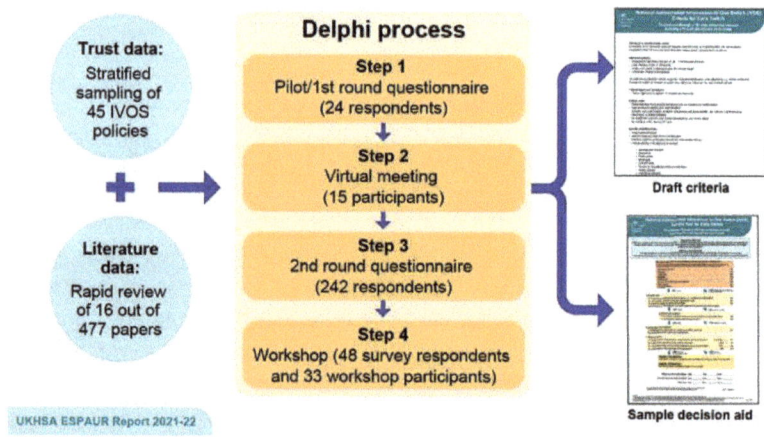

Figure 2. Development of a national intravenous-to-oral switch (IVOS) criteria for use in secondary care.

IVOS criteria from forty-five policies and 16 (out of 477 papers identified from the literature search) led to a collated list of 41 IVOS criteria. These were subsequently formatted into 5-point Likert scale questions for Step 1) pilot/1st round questionnaire. Step 2) virtual meeting, accepted 36 IVOS criteria for inclusion in Step 3). Step 3) 2nd round questionnaire. So far, 86% of 2nd round questionnaire respondents (n = 169) agree/strongly agree that a patient's early warning score should be improving for a safe and effective IVOS. The final criteria will be published as part of UKHSA's AMR guidance and regulation collection webpage [8].

4. Conclusions

Developing and implementing AMS strategies across healthcare sectors is vital to tackle the global health threat that is AMR. In primary care, evidenced-based tools were developed for clinicians to support addressing high rates of long-term and repeat prescribing in acne and COPD exacerbations. During 2022–2023, the national AMS toolkit for primary care, the TARGET Antibiotics Toolkit website, was updated with new resources to support antibiotics discussions with patients, and there are plans to develop resources for common skin infections. In secondary care, the consensus is being defined for a UK-wide criteria and tool to support prompt antimicrobial IV to oral switch decisions.

Author Contributions: Conceptualization, D.A.-O., S.P. and D.L.; methodology, E.C. (Ella Casale), D.A.-O., C.V.H., D.L., L.O., E.S., E.C. (Emily Cooper), F.P., S.P. and E.J.H.; formal analysis, C.V.H. and E.J.H.; data curation, C.V.H., L.O., E.S., E.C., F.P., S.P. and E.J.H.; writing—original draft preparation, E.C. (Ella Casale), C.V.H., E.J.H., E.C. (Emily Cooper), E.S. and L.O.; writing—review and editing, E.C. (Emily Cooper), D.A.-O., C.V.H., D.L., L.O., E.S., E.C. (Emily Cooper), F.P., S.P. and E.J.H.; supervision, D.A.-O. and D.L.; funding acquisition, D.A.-O., S.P. and D.L. All authors have read and agreed to the published version of the manuscript.

Funding: This research received no external funding.

Institutional Review Board Statement: Not applicable.

Informed Consent Statement: Not applicable.

Data Availability Statement: Full data are available in this year's ESPAUR report [3].

Acknowledgments: We would like to thank Alex Orlek, Louise Fisher, and Brian MacKenna for their contributions to the analysis of the OpenSafely data and to Jon White for creating the infographics. The authors would also like to acknowledge the ESPAUR Oversight Group members.

Conflicts of Interest: The authors declare no conflict of interest.

References

1. Tackling Antimicrobial Resistance 2019 to 2024: The UK's 5-Year National Action Plan. Available online: https://www.gov.uk/government/publications/uk-5-year-action-plan-for-antimicrobial-resistance-2019-to-2024 (accessed on 20 August 2022).
2. Ashiru-Oredope, D.; Hopkins, S.; on behalf of the English Surveillance Programme for Antimicrobial Utilization and Resistance Oversight Group; Kessel, A.; Hopkins, S.; Ashiru-Oredope, D.; Brown, B.; Brown, N.; Carter, S.; Charlett, A.; et al. Antimicrobial stewardship: English surveillance programme for antimicrobial utilization and resistance (ESPAUR). *J. Antimicrob. Chemother.* **2013**, *68*, 2421–2423. [CrossRef] [PubMed]
3. Hayes, C.; Casale, E.; Lecky, D.; O'Neil, L.; Sides, E.; Cooper, E.; Pursey, F.; Pa-rekh, S.; Fisher, L.; MacKenna, B.; et al. Chapter 4 Antimicrobial Stewardship. In *English Surveillance Programme for Antimicrobial Utilisation and Resistance (ESPAUR) Report 2021 to 2022*; UK Health Security Agency: London, UK, 2022.
4. TARGET Antibiotics Toolkit Hub. Available online: https://elearning.rcgp.org.uk/course/view.php?id=553.2022 (accessed on 15 August 2022).
5. TARGET Antibiotics Toolkit Hub-Leaflets to Discuss with Patients. Available online: https://elearning.rcgp.org.uk/mod/book/view.php?id=12647 (accessed on 15 August 2022).
6. TARGET Antibiotics Toolkit Hub–Resources for the Community Pharmacy Setting. Available online: https://elearning.rcgp.org.uk/mod/book/view.php?id=13511 (accessed on 15 August 2022).
7. The Community Pharmacy Contractual Framework for 2019/20 to 2023/24: Supporting Delivery for the NHS Long Term Plan. Available online: https://www.gov.uk/government/publications/community-pharmacy-contractual-framework-2019-to-2024 (accessed on 15 August 2022).
8. Antimicrobial Resistance: Guidance and Regulation Collection. Available online: https://www.gov.uk/health-and-social-care/antimicrobial-resistance (accessed on 15 August 2022).

Disclaimer/Publisher's Note: The statements, opinions and data contained in all publications are solely those of the individual author(s) and contributor(s) and not of MDPI and/or the editor(s). MDPI and/or the editor(s) disclaim responsibility for any injury to people or property resulting from any ideas, methods, instructions or products referred to in the content.

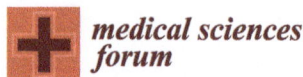 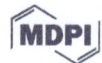

Proceeding Paper

Antimicrobial Resistance: Professional and Public Education, Engagement, and Training Activities 2021–2022 (ESPAUR Report) †

Catherine V. Hayes [1,*], Jordan Charlesworth [1], Diane Ashiru-Oredope [1], Eirwen Sides [1], Amy Jackson [1], Emily Cooper [1], Brieze Read [1], Donna Seaton [2], Lorna Flintham [2], Harpreet Sidhu [3] and Donna M. Lecky [1,*]

1. HCAI, Fungal, AMR, AMU & Sepsis Division, UK Health Security Agency, London SW1P 3JR, UK; diane.ashiru-oredope@ukhsa.gov.uk (D.A.-O.)
2. Faculty of Biology, Medicine and Health, University of Manchester, Manchester M13 9PL, UK
3. Department of Pharmacy, Aston University, Aston St, Birmingham B4 7ET, UK
* Correspondence: catherine.hayes@ukhsa.gov.uk (C.V.H.); donna.lecky@ukhsa.gov.uk (D.M.L.)
† Presented at the ESPAUR 2021/22 Webinar, Antibiotic Guardian, 23 November 2022; Available online: https://antibioticguardian.com/Meetings/espaur-2021-22-webinar/.

Abstract: This is a summary of initiatives to engage and educate the general public and healthcare professionals about antimicrobial use, stewardship and resistance, as covered in the 2021–2022 English Surveillance Programme for Antimicrobial Utilisation and Resistance (ESPAUR) Report. Activities led by the UK Health Security Agency (UKHSA) and collaborating organisations are highlighted.

Keywords: antimicrobial resistance; antimicrobial stewardship; schools; primary care; community pharmacy; secondary care; general practice; continuing professional development

1. Introduction

The education and engagement of healthcare professionals (HCPs) and the public are crucial to antimicrobial stewardship (AMS), and are highlighted in the UK 20-year vision for tackling antimicrobial resistance (AMR) and the 5-year National Action Plan (NAP) [1,2]. The COVID-19 pandemic significantly disrupted education and training. However, as social restrictions eased, there was renewed vigour for professional and public education, engagement, and training. This paper summarizes Chapter 6 of the annual English Surveillance Programme for Antimicrobial Utilisation and Resistance (ESPAUR) report, detailing the UKHSA-led education and training activities in England from 2021 to 2022 [3,4]. These findings were presented at the ESPAUR Report webinar on 23 November 2022.

2. Healthcare Professional Training

Remote learning, established during the COVID-19 pandemic, continued across all sectors for the training of HCPs, including online training modules, online conferences, and webinars. Training focused on renewing key AMS messages across the patient pathway, using the TARGET Antibiotic Toolkit resources [5] and discussing antibiotics with patients. There is currently no mandatory training on AMS for HCPs.

3. Public and Professional Engagement

The Antibiotic Guardian (AG) campaign [6] engages professionals and the public to pledge to help keep antibiotics working. Since launching in 2014 to the end of 2021, there were 144,446 pledges on the main AG webpage (Figure 1). A total of 65% of all pledges were made by those identifying as a health/social care professional or leader, and of these, 72% were from pharmacy teams (including primary and secondary care and community pharmacies).

Citation: Hayes, C.V.; Charlesworth, J.; Ashiru-Oredope, D.; Sides, E.; Jackson, A.; Cooper, E.; Read, B.; Seaton, D.; Flintham, L.; Sidhu, H.; et al. Antimicrobial Resistance: Professional and Public Education, Engagement, and Training Activities 2021–2022 (ESPAUR Report). *Med. Sci. Forum* **2022**, *15*, 19. https://doi.org/10.3390/msf2022015019

Academic Editor: Vanessa Carter

Published: 5 July 2023

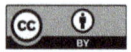

Copyright: © 2023 by the authors. Licensee MDPI, Basel, Switzerland. This article is an open access article distributed under the terms and conditions of the Creative Commons Attribution (CC BY) license (https://creativecommons.org/licenses/by/4.0/).

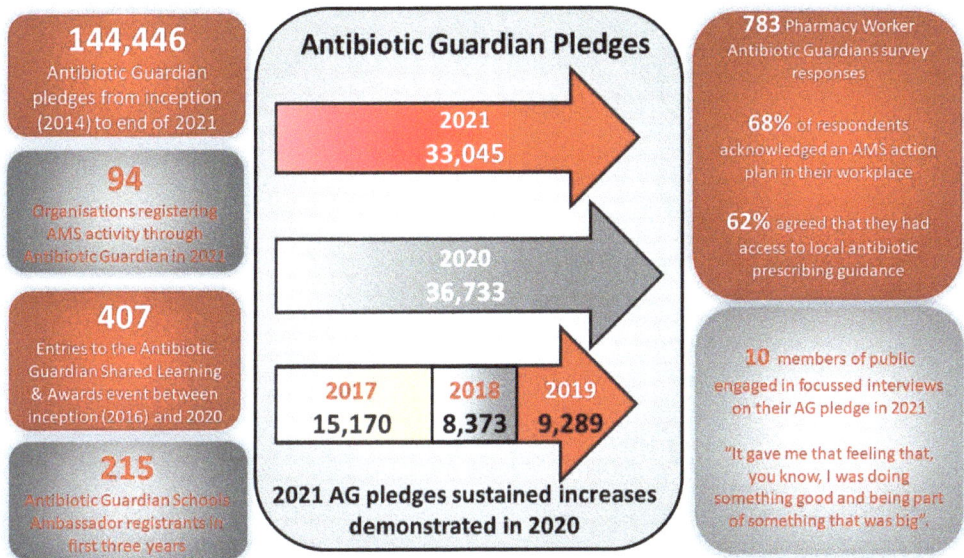

Figure 1. An infographic summarising Antibiotic Guardian pledge activity between 2017 and the end of 2021, alongside information on Antibiotic Guardian-related activity. Infographic adapted with permission from Ref. [4]. Copyright 2022 UK Health Security Agency.

An evaluation of the AG campaign focused on the public and pharmacy workers. A survey of pharmacy workers identified statistically significant differences in the AMS capability of different roles across the pharmacy profession [7]. Qualitative interviews with the public who had pledged to be an Antibiotic Guardian identified motivations based on moral obligation, personal responsibility, and uncertainty about the future.

The Antibiotic Guardian School Ambassadors programme was first piloted in 2019 and connects HCPs with local schools and community groups to educate people about AMR. A total of 110 colleagues registered in 2021, and pharmacists have been accounted for the most volunteers each year. Ambassadors reported the personal and professional benefits of participating.

World Antimicrobial Awareness Week (WAAW) and the European Antimicrobial Awareness Day (EAAD) 2021 aimed to engage HCPs and the public on tackling AMR. Continuing the precedent set during the COVID-19 pandemic, the campaign was mainly digital, focusing on sharing information via social media and digital notes. Twitter activity during WAAW 2021 included 15,452 tweets from 6189 users, and 37,719 retweets from 17,808 users during the week.

4. Public Engagement

The e-Bug programme [8], operated by UKHSA, provides educational resources to support children and young people (aged 3–16 years) in all communities with information on infection prevention and AMR topics (see Figure 2). The e-Bug educational resources underwent a full review and update, and with support from NHS England, they were disseminated to every maintained school and academy across England (over 20,000 schools) in January 2022. See Figure 3 for more detail on e-Bug activities.

Infographic 27. e-Bug achievements

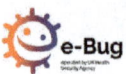

From 2021 to 22, the e-Bug programme has:

 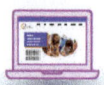 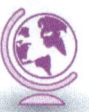

Developed educational resources with teachers and scientists for ages 3-16. These are mapped to the National Curriculum and accredited by the Association for Science Education

Disseminated educational resources to **20,318** primary and secondary schools across England

Launched an interim website (www.e-bug.eu) to share the resources, receiving **520,914** page views from **214** countries

Raised awareness amongst the public. Shared **175** tweets creating **156,381** impressions, and presented at **4** conferences to over **6000** attendees

Collaborated with **17** countries to highlight the importance of including education of children and young people in AMR strategies

UKHSA ESPAUR Report 2021-22

Figure 2. Infection prevention and AMR topics covered in the e-Bug educational resources. Infographic adapted with permission from Ref. [4]. Copyright 2022 UK Health Security Agency.

Infographic 28. e-Bug: supporting children and young people

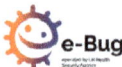

Across the e-Bug resources, children and young people are supported to:

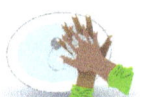 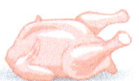 

Embed hygiene practices to prevent the spread of infection

Adopt safe preparation and cooking practices to avoid food-borne illness

Understand what microbes are and that antibiotics only work for bacteria

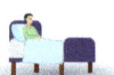 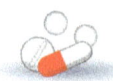

Adopt self-care methods when appropriate

Only take antimicrobials as and when prescribed

Grow up as antimicrobial stewards

UKHSA ESPAUR Report 2021-22

Figure 3. e-Bug programme activities from 2021 to 2022. Infographic adapted with permission from Ref. [4]. Copyright 2022 UK Health Security Agency.

5. Conclusions

Future work in public and professional education includes plans for a national implementation of TARGET and e-Bug training and resources, aiming for the consistent education of HCPs and the public in the future.

Author Contributions: Conceptualization, D.M.L. and D.A-O.; methodology, C.V.H., J.C., D.A-O., E.S.; A.J.; E.C.; B.R., D.S., L.F., H.S. and D.M.L.; formal analysis, C.V.H., J.C., E.S., A.J., E.C., B.R., D.S., L.F. and H.S.; data curation, C.V.H., J.C., E.S., A.J., E.C., B.R., D.S., L.F. and H.S.; writing—original draft preparation, C.V.H., J.C., E.S., A.J., E.C., B.R., D.S., L.F. and H.S.; writing—review and editing, C.V.H., J.C., D.A.-O., E.S., A.J., E.C., B.R., D.S., L.F., H.S. and D.M.L.; supervision, D.M.L. and D.A.-O. All authors have read and agreed to the published version of the manuscript.

Funding: This research received no external funding.

Institutional Review Board Statement: Not applicable.

Informed Consent Statement: Not applicable.

Data Availability Statement: Full data are available in this year's ESPAUR report [4].

Acknowledgments: Thank you to contributors: Fionna Pursey, Magda Hann, Claire Neill, Marzena Edwards, Gillian Hayes, Rose Hadden, Sarah Tonkin-Crine, Monsey MacLeod, Rabia Ahmed, Roger Harrison, Isla Gemmell, Elizabeth Dalgarno, and Jon White for creating the infographics. The authors would like to acknowledge the ESPAUR Oversight Group members.

Conflicts of Interest: The authors declare no conflict of interest.

References

1. *UK 5-Year Action Plan for Antimicrobial Resistance 2019 to 2024*; Department of Health and Social Care: London, UK, 2019.
2. *UK 20-Year Vision for Antimicrobial Resistance*; Department of Health and Social Care: London, UK, 2019.
3. Ashiru-Oredope, D.; Hopkins, S.; on behalf of the English Surveillance Programme for Antimicrobial Utilization and Resistance Oversight Group. Antimicrobial stewardship: English surveillance programme for antimicrobial utilization and resistance (ESPAUR). *J. Antimicrob. Chemother.* **2013**, *68*, 2421–2423. [CrossRef] [PubMed]
4. Hayes, C.V.; Charlesworth, J.; Ashiru-Oredope, D.; Sides, E.; Jackson, A.; Cooper, E.; Read, B.; Seaton, D.; Flintham, L.; Sidhu, H.; et al. Chapter 6 Professional and public education, engagement, and training. In *The English Surveillance Programme for Antimicrobial Utilisation and Resistance (ESPAUR) Report 2021 to 2022*; UK Health Security Agency: London, UK, 2022.
5. Royal College of General Practitioners. TARGET Antibiotics Toolkit Hub. Available online: https://elearning.rcgp.org.uk/course/view.php?id=553 (accessed on 15 August 2022).
6. Antibiotic Guardian. Available online: https://antibioticguardian.com (accessed on 19 October 2022).
7. Seaton, D.; Ashiru-Oredope, D.; Charlesworth, J.; Gemmell, I.; Harrison, R. Evaluating UK Pharmacy Workers' Knowledge, Attitudes and Behaviour towards Antimicrobial Stewardship and Assessing the Impact of Training in Community Pharmacy. *Pharmacy* **2022**, *10*, 98. [CrossRef] [PubMed]
8. e-Bug. Available online: https://e-Bug.eu (accessed on 19 October 2022).

Disclaimer/Publisher's Note: The statements, opinions and data contained in all publications are solely those of the individual author(s) and contributor(s) and not of MDPI and/or the editor(s). MDPI and/or the editor(s) disclaim responsibility for any injury to people or property resulting from any ideas, methods, instructions or products referred to in the content.

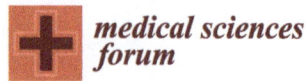
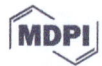

Proceeding Paper

Surveillance and Stewardship Approaches for COVID-19 Novel Therapeutics in England from 2021 to 2022 (ESPAUR Report) †

Alessandra Løchen [1,*], Hanna Squire [1], Diane Ashiru-Oredope [1], Kieran S. Hand [2], Hassan Hartman [1], Carry Triggs-Hodge [1], Holly Fountain [1], Sabine Bou-Antoun [1], Alicia Demirjian [1,3,4] and Sarah M. Gerver [1,*]

1. United Kingdom Health Security Agency (UKHSA), London NW9 5EQ, UK
2. Medical Directorate, NHS England, London SE1 8UG, UK
3. Department of Paediatric Infectious Diseases and Immunology, Evelina London Children's Hospital, London SE1 7EH, UK
4. Faculty of Life Sciences and Medicine, King's College London, London WC2R 2LS, UK
* Correspondence: alessandra.lochen@ukhsa.gov.uk (A.L.); sarah.gerver@ukhsa.gov.uk (S.M.G.)
† Presented at the ESPAUR 2021/22 Webinar, Antibiotic Guardian, 23 November 2022; Available online: https://antibioticguardian.com/Meetings/espaur-2021-22-webinar/.

Abstract: The UK Health Security Agency's (UKHSA) COVID-19 therapeutics programme was commissioned by the Department of Health and Social Care with the remit to evaluate the use and role of COVID-19 treatments. COVID-19 therapeutics data were assessed from two main data sources: novel therapy requests via Blueteq and medicines supply data via Rx-info. The five COVID-19 therapies in use in England between 1 October 2021 and 31 March 2022 included nirmatrelvir plus ritonavir, remdesivir, molnupiravir, sotrovimab, and casirivimab with imdevimab. During this time period, treatment requests for novel therapies against COVID-19 were submitted for nearly 52,000 patients in England. The UKHSAs COVID-19 therapeutics programme has been key to supporting the deployment of novel COVID-19 therapies in England by undertaking genomic, virological, and epidemiologic surveillance, through both national surveillance systems and academic collaboration. Effective therapies are particularly important for protecting the health of patients at greater risk of developing severe COVID-19. This national surveillance and stewardship programme was successfully rolled out at pace at the start of the pandemic and leads on work nationally to reduce the development of resistance. These findings were presented at the ESPAUR Report webinar on 23 November 2022.

Keywords: COVID-19 novel therapeutics; neutralising monoclonal antibodies; antivirals; COVID-19; antimicrobial stewardship

Citation: Løchen, A.; Squire, H.; Ashiru-Oredope, D.; Hand, K.S.; Hartman, H.; Triggs-Hodge, C.; Fountain, H.; Bou-Antoun, S.; Demirjian, A.; Gerver, S.M. Surveillance and Stewardship Approaches for COVID-19 Novel Therapeutics in England from 2021 to 2022 (ESPAUR Report). *Med. Sci. Forum* **2022**, *15*, 2. https://doi.org/10.3390/msf2022015002

Academic Editor: Alan Johnson

Published: 1 March 2023

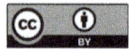

Copyright: © 2023 by the authors. Licensee MDPI, Basel, Switzerland. This article is an open access article distributed under the terms and conditions of the Creative Commons Attribution (CC BY) license (https://creativecommons.org/licenses/by/4.0/).

1. Introduction

In March 2020, the World Health Organisation (WHO) declared coronavirus disease 2019 (COVID-19) caused by severe acute respiratory syndrome coronavirus 2 (SARS-CoV-2) a Public Health Emergency of International Concern. Coordinated international efforts identified therapeutic candidates to treat severe illness from COVID-19, and since late 2020, England has had five direct-acting antiviral agents added to the clinical commissioning policy. These were three antivirals: nirmatrelvir plus ritonavir (Paxlovid), remdesivir (Veklury), and molnupiravir (Lagevrio), and two neutralising monoclonal antibody therapies (nMAbs): sotrovimab (Xevudy) and casirivimab with imdevimab (Ronapreve). The annual English Surveillance Programme for Antimicrobial Utilisation and Resistance (ESPAUR) report, Chapter 7, commentates on the UK Health Security Agency's (UKHSA) COVID-19 therapeutics programme [1,2].

2. Methods

The UKHSA COVID-19 therapeutics programme was commissioned by the Department of Health and Social Care with the remit and objective to evaluate the use and role of COVID-19 treatments. COVID-19 therapeutics data were assessed from two main data sources: Blueteq and Rx-info. The Blueteq system supports the management of high-cost drugs for NHS England and, as such, contains clinical requests made for neutralising monoclonal antibodies (nMAB) and antiviral therapies used for the treatment of patients with COVID-19 who fall in the remit of the clinical commissioning policy. Not all treatment requests may have resulted in patients receiving treatment with these drugs; this is the most informative data source in the absence of patient-level prescribing data. The Rx-info data contain medicines supply data from all NHS acute hospital Trusts, including standardised transactional data on the procurement, stock-holding, and issuing of medicines by NHS Trusts, and therefore provides a picture of the total usage of COVID-19 therapeutics in England. COVID-19 therapeutics treatment requests were extracted from the Blueteq system on 22 August 2022 and medicines supply data in England via Rx-info on 12 June 2022, for the period 1 October 2021 to 31 March 2022, was inclusive and covered the five direct-acting antiviral agents in use in England during this period. The date of treatment recorded in the Blueteq data was used for treatment requests. Not all of these therapeutic agents were available throughout the whole period (Figure 1).

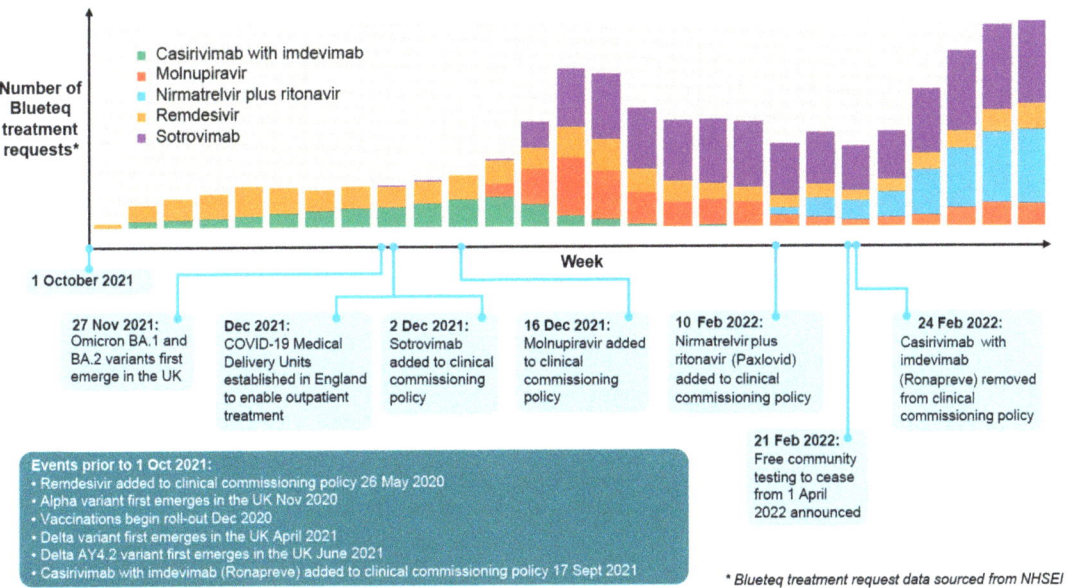

Figure 1. COVID-19 therapeutic Blueteq treatment requests by week (1 October 2021 to 31 March 2022) and a timeline of events.

Data from Blueteq patient treatment requests were cleaned (for non-approved entries, invalid NHS numbers, or duplicate entries) and linked to demographic, vaccination (National Immunisation Management Service [NIMS] dataset), hospital stay (Emergency Care Dataset and Secondary Uses Service (SUS) hospital data, the spell during which the patient received therapy), mortality data (as described in [3]), and viral genomic and mutations data, to provide patient-level epidemiological data on the use of these new therapeutic agents and the patients treated in England. Data were deterministically linked using NHS number. Treatment requests data were at the patient level.

Rx-info data captured the number of medicines dispensed daily (Virtual Medicinal Product [VMP] quantity in daily dispensed grams), and the use of these key therapies by NHS acute Trusts and regionally is described in [2]).

At the time of compiling this report, data on the number of patients eligible to receive COVID-19 therapeutics were unavailable to UKHSA, and so population data taken from the Office of National Statistics annual mid-year population estimates and number of persons with COVID-19 in that group over the specified period were used as denominators for rate calculations.

Comparisons of treated patients (Blueteq treatment requests) and medicines supplied (Rx-info medicine supply data) were completed by calculating the total grams of nMABs and antivirals that have an approved Blueteq request form (estimated from expected duration and dose) against the grams dispensed from Rx-info. Standardised doses for each therapy were used to calculate Rx-info usage [2]. The differences in grams between the two sources was calculated to highlight discrepancies in the total medicines supply and treatment requests. This analysis was completed for England, and also by NHS region, taking into account the stock provided to centres.

STATA 15 was used in all medicines supply data analysis. R was used in all other analyses.

3. Results

3.1. Treatment Requests (BlueTeq data)

Between 1 October and 31 March 2022, 51,962 treatment requests for neutralising monoclonal antibodies and antivirals against COVID-19 were made in England. Of these, sotrovimab had the highest number of treatment requests and made up almost 38% (n = 19,749 requests) of all English treatment requests.

The usage of COVID-19 therapies varies by age, sex, ethnicity, NHS region, and index of multiple deprivation (IMD). Overall request rates have shown a large range between NHS England regions (Table 1). The east of England had the highest rate of treatment requests per 100,000 population and per 100,000 COVID-19 cases; these accounted for approximately twice those observed in the northwest. In addition, the southeast, while having a higher treatment request rate per 100,000 population than the northeast and Yorkshire, had a lower rate per 100,000 COVID-19 cases. Regional differences in the establishment of COVID-19 Medical Delivery Units, responsible for outpatient treatment, and in the COVID-19 case rates, may have impacted the treatment rates per 100,000 COVID-19 cases. These findings highlight regional variations in COVID-19 reported cases that may impact treatment request rates.

Table 1. Number, percentage, and rate (per 100,000 population and per 100,000 COVID-19 cases) of treatment requests in Blueteq by NHS Region between 1 October 2021 and 31 March 2022.

NHS Region	No. Requests	Percent	Rates per 100,000 Population	Rates per 100,000 COVID-19 Cases
East of England	7967	15%	121.4	589.1
London	9910	19%	110.1	587.5
Southwest	6018	12%	106.2	522.8
Southeast	8161	16%	91.3	436.2
Northeast and Yorkshire	7115	14%	82.4	447.3
Midlands	8552	16%	80.2	433.7
Northwest	4178	8%	58.9	311.7

While differences exist in the number of treatment requests between males and females in corresponding age groups, males and females did not differ significantly in the rate of treatment requests per 100,000 COVID-19 cases in age–sex categories.

The breakdown in therapeutic agent requests by ethnicity, despite small numbers in some ethnic groups, indicates a divergence in treatment choice between the White, Indian, and Mixed ethnic groups compared to the Black, Pakistani, and Other Asian groups. While the distribution of treatment requests is comparable between the White, Indian, and Mixed ethnic groups, a larger percentage of treatment requests for the Black, Pakistani, and other Asian groups are for remdesivir (over 30% compared to 18–20% for these other ethnic groups). Sotrovimab makes up less than 30% of requests in the Black group compared to White, Indian, and mixed ethnic groups, where it makes up 40–47% of requests.

When assessed by IMD decile, treatments commonly used in the community, such as nirmatrelvir plus ritonavir and sotrovimab, have a higher percentage of requests for patients from the most deprived areas compared to those from the least deprived areas, whereas treatments commonly administered in hospitals, such as remdesivir and casirivimab with imdevimab, show the reverse pattern.

3.2. Comparison of Treatment Requests with Rx-Info Medicines Supply Data

For all COVID-19 therapeutics, there was an apparent excess of grams dispensed according to Rx-info data compared to the grams expected from Blueteq requests for all months where the therapy was in use. Remdesivir generally had the highest percentage of excess Rx-info use (ranging 45–59% across the months it was in use), whereas sotrovimab (16–26%) and nirmatrelvir plus ritonavir (21–23%) had the lowest range of excess Rx-info usage across the months they were in use.

3.3. Genomic Surveillance

Treatment-emergent SARS-CoV-2 mutations were screened for by comparing the sequenced samples from patients before (>5000) and after treatment (>1400) and identifying significant changes in mutation frequencies between the pre- and post-treatment samples. The analysis was stratified by treatment and variant and yielded eleven mutations from Delta samples treated with casirivimab with imdevimab, BA.1 and BA.2 samples treated with sotrovimab, and Alpha samples treated with remdesivir [1].

4. Discussion

The UKHSAs COVID-19 therapeutics programme has supported the deployment of novel COVID-19 therapies in England by undertaking genomic, virological, and epidemiological surveillance and stewardship approaches, through both national surveillance systems and academic collaboration. Effective therapies are particularly important for protecting the health of patients at greater risk of developing severe COVID-19. Genomic surveillance has allowed for the rapid identification of mutations and variants associated with a resistance to certain therapeutics. This national surveillance and stewardship programme was successfully rolled out at pace at the start of the pandemic and contributes to work nationally to reduce the development of resistance. The programme has provided an evidence base to guide clinical commissioning policies for COVID-19 therapeutics. For example, epidemiological surveillance directly informed national discussions on the use of sotrovimab for the treatment of Omicron BA.1 versus BA.2 after the US Food and Drug Administration removed the therapy for use against Omicron BA.2 based on laboratory analyses. This helped ensure that patients were receiving the most effective treatments available.

Absolute numbers of treatment requests from Blueteq showed variation by NHS region, age, sex, ethnicity, and IMD by therapeutic agent, although denominator data were not available for each subgroup. Therapeutic treatment requests largely followed the trends that would be expected within the context of the setting they were administered in. For instance, remdesivir, which is commonly used in the hospital setting, had more treatment requests during the Delta wave than the Delta sublineagee AY4.2 wave, as the Delta variant had higher hospitalisation rates. Furthermore, a divergence in the crude number of treatment requests by intervention and by setting between certain ethnic groups and between the least versus most deprived groups highlights the need to explore differential access by way of comparison using a denominator dataset with the total eligible population. Overall, the interpretation of the work presented here is limited as it uses the overall population; therefore, differences between sub-populations merit further exploration to understand whether they are significant based on treatment eligibility. This highlights the need for the work that NHSE conducts, through its NHS Foundry platform and beyond, to rapidly deploy antiviral agents and manage operational delivery and performance, complemented by UKHSAs therapeutic surveillance.

One key finding on the usage of COVID-19 therapies is that there is a discrepancy between the treatment requests (Blueteq) and the medicines supply data (Rx-info). Whereas Blueteq captures patient-level applications for the renumeration of high-cost medicines, Rx-info captures stock movements within hospital pharmacies and potentially provides a more comprehensive picture of usage. The use of standardised doses for Rx-info data may account for some of the discrepancies between BlueTeq and Rx-info usage where varying doses or treatment durations are used in practice. Despite these limitations, the addition of the Blueteq system to the toolkit of antimicrobial resistance is a helpful and welcome one and can be used as a blueprint for the roll out of new antimicrobial agents in the future.

Author Contributions: Methodology, S.M.G., A.D., D.A.-O., S.B.-A. and A.L.; formal analysis, A.L., H.S., H.H. and H.F.; writing—original draft preparation, A.L., H.S., D.A.-O., K.S.H., H.H., C.T.-H., H.F., S.B.-A., A.D. and S.M.G.; writing—review and editing, A.L., H.S., D.A.-O., K.S.H., H.H., C.T.-H., H.F., S.B.-A., A.D. and S.M.G.; supervision, S.M.G., A.D. and D.A.-O. All authors have read and agreed to the published version of the manuscript.

Funding: This research received no external funding.

Institutional Review Board Statement: Not applicable.

Informed Consent Statement: Patient consent was not sought under Section 251 of the National Health Service Act 2006 permits UKHSA use of patient-level data for specific projects.

Data Availability Statement: The data presented in this study are available in [Squire, H.; Lochen, A.; Ashiru-Oredope, D.; Hand, K. S.; Hartman, H.; Triggs-Hodge, C.; Fountain, H.; Bou-Antoun, S.; Gerver, S.; Demirjian, A. Chapter 7 COVID-19 therapeutics. In *English Surveillance Programme for Antimicrobial Utilisation and Resistance (ESPAUR) Report 2021 to 2022*; UK Health Security Agency: London, UK, 2022].

Acknowledgments: Sakib Rokadiya, Manon Ragonnet, Gareth Arthur, Ann Jarvis, Phillip Howard, Bethan Davies, Susan Hopkins, Colin Brown. The authors would like to acknowledge the ESPAUR Oversight Group members.

Conflicts of Interest: The authors declare no conflict of interest.

References

1. Ashiru-Oredope, D.; Hopkins, S.; on behalf of the English Surveillance Programme for Antimicrobial Utilization and Resistance Oversight Group; Kessel, A.; Hopkins, S.; Ashiru-Oredope, D.; Brown, B.; Brown, N.; Carter, S.; Charlett, A.; et al. Antimicrobial stewardship: English surveillance programme for antimicrobial utilization and resistance (ESPAUR). *J. Antimicrob. Chemother.* **2013**, *68*, 2421–2425. [CrossRef] [PubMed]
2. Squire, H.; Lochen, A.; Ashiru-Oredope, D.; Hand, K.; Hartman, H.; Triggs-Hodge, C.; Fountain, H.; Bou-Antoun, S.; Gerver, S.; Demirjian, A. Chapter 7 COVID-19 therapeutics. In *English Surveillance Programme for Antimicrobial Utilisation and Resistance (ESPAUR) Report 2021 to 2022*; UK Health Security Agency: London, UK, 2022.
3. Twohig, K.A.; Nyberg, T.; Zaidi, A.; Thelwall, S.; Sinnathamby, M.A.; Aliabadi, M.; Seaman, S.R.; Harris, R.J.; Hope, R.; Lopez-Bernal, J.; et al. Hospital admission and emergency care attendance risk for SARS-CoV-2 delta (B.1.617.2) compared with alpha (B.1.1.7) variants of concern: A cohort study. *Lancet Infect. Dis.* **2022**, *22*, 35–42. [CrossRef] [PubMed]

Disclaimer/Publisher's Note: The statements, opinions and data contained in all publications are solely those of the individual author(s) and contributor(s) and not of MDPI and/or the editor(s). MDPI and/or the editor(s) disclaim responsibility for any injury to people or property resulting from any ideas, methods, instructions or products referred to in the content.

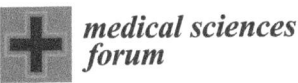

Abstract

Research on Antimicrobial Utilization and Resistance in England 2021–22 (ESPAUR Report) [†]

Emily Agnew * and Julie V. Robotham * on behalf of the ESPAUR Research Chapter Authors

HCAI & AMR Modelling and Evaluation Unit, HCAI, Fungal, AMR, AMU & Sepsis Division, Clinical and Public Health Group, UK Health Security Agency, 61 Colindale Avenue, London NW9 5EQ, UK

* Correspondence: emily.agnew@ukhsa.gov.uk (E.A.); julie.robotham@ukhsa.gov.uk (J.V.R)
† Presented at the Antibiotic Guardian 2022 Shared Learning & Awards; Available online: https://antibioticguardian.com/antibiotic-guardian-2022-shared-learning-awards/.

Keywords: ESPAUR Report; research; antimicrobial resistance; UK Health Security Agency

Citation: Agnew, E.; Robotham, J.V. Research on Antimicrobial Utilization and Resistance in England 2021–22 (ESPAUR Report). *Med. Sci. Forum* **2022**, *15*, 17. https://doi.org/10.3390/msf2022015017

Published: 28 March 2023

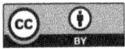

Copyright: © 2023 by the authors. Licensee MDPI, Basel, Switzerland. This article is an open access article distributed under the terms and conditions of the Creative Commons Attribution (CC BY) license (https://creativecommons.org/licenses/by/4.0/).

The Research Chapter (Chapter 8) of the English Surveillance Programme for Antimicrobial Utilisation and Resistance (ESPAUR) Report 2021–2022 showcases the research that has been undertaken and that is ongoing at the UK Health Security Agency (UKHSA) in the field of healthcare-associated infections (HCAIs) and antimicrobial resistance (AMR) from April 2021 to March 2022 [1,2]. These findings were presented at the ESPAUR Report webinar on 23 November 2022.

This chapter highlights the scope and breadth of projects that are underway covering many research and development priorities, including improvements in surveillance and data collection and enhancing insights drawn from them. Work has been directed to the development of novel diagnostics and treatments, as well as improving the evidence base for existing control strategies, including infection prevention and control (IPC), antimicrobial stewardship (AMS), diagnostics, antimicrobials, and novel alternatives (such as vaccination and host-directed therapies). A significant amount of research has been undertaken to improve our understanding of the mechanisms of disease transmission, risk factors for carriage and infection, and the health and economic burden. As well as covering a breadth of topic areas, this research also uses a breadth of methodologies, both quantitative and qualitative, from mathematical modelling to behavioral research, and from exploratory laboratory science to implementation science. The projects covered in the chapter span the majority of the major themes of the national action plan (NAP) for AMR [3], as shown in Figure 1.

Examples of AMR and HCAI research projects from across the NAP's major themes are described in the chapter, with the majority of projects reflecting the themes of 'Stronger laboratory capacity and surveillance in AMR', 'Human infection prevention and control', and the 'Optimal use of antimicrobials'. Further projects cover the themes of 'Basic research', the 'Development of new therapeutics', and 'Development and access to novel diagnostics'. The publication distribution in Figure 2 shows that there is also cutting-edge research underway across the following topics: 'Environmental contamination', 'Better food safety', 'Wider access to therapeutics', 'Development and access to vaccines', 'Better quality assurance', and 'International diplomacy'.

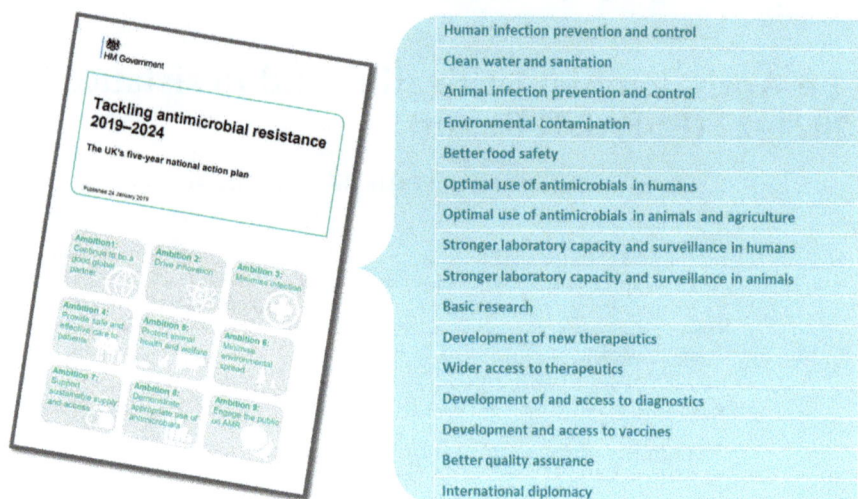

Figure 1. National action plan major AMR themes. Adapted from Ref. [3].

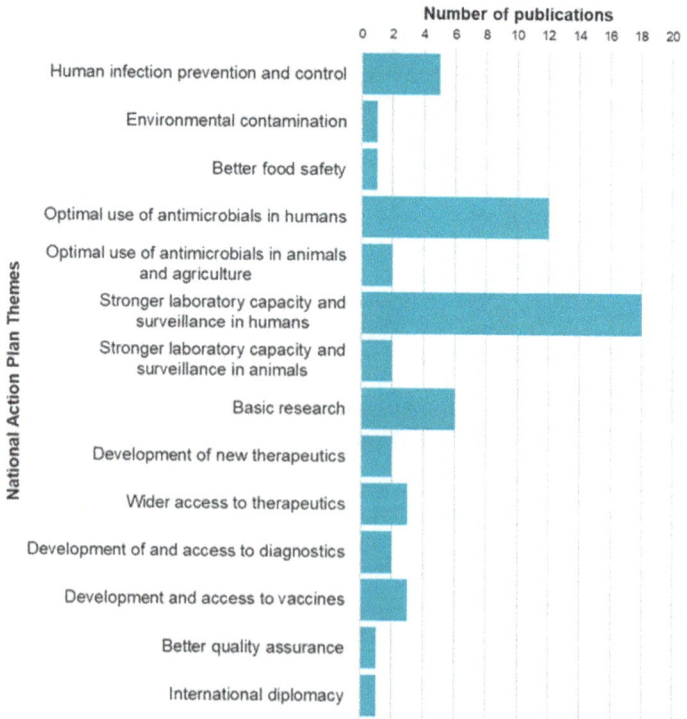

Figure 2. An illustration of the wide distribution of almost 60 publications [4–61] from UKHSA across the NAP's major themes.

Research from the two National Institute for Health Research (NIHR) Health Protection Research Units (HPRUs) in the topic areas of HCAI and AMR, led by Imperial College London and Oxford University in partnership with UKHSA, is highlighted. The HPRUs are multi-disciplinary centers of excellence, with a focus on collaboration, training, and knowledge sharing. An overview of the four main research themes of each HCAI and AMR

HPRU is provided and individual exemplar research projects are described, demonstrating the breadth and scale of the work within the HPRUs. These include, for example, a large-scale observational hybrid sequencing-based study that explores the mobilomes associated with Gram-negative bloodstream infections, and work in collaboration with global expert stakeholders to develop a research roadmap for optimizing antibiotic use in human populations. The work of HPRUs is intended to be translational, e.g., helping to shape the next national action plan. As such, in unity with the goals of HPRUs, this chapter highlights the importance of—and approaches to— embedding knowledge mobilization, optimizing the use of research-generated knowledge, and ensuring that the right audiences are reached in the right way to achieve the greatest impact.

Author Contributions: Writing—original draft preparation, E.A. and J.V.R.; writing—review and editing, E.A. and J.V.R. All authors have read and agreed to the published version of the manuscript.

Funding: This research received no external funding.

Institutional Review Board Statement: Not applicable.

Informed Consent Statement: Not applicable.

Data Availability Statement: Data sharing not applicable.

Acknowledgments: We acknowledge the contribution of the all of the authors of the ESPAUR research chapter: Jordan Charlesworth, Joanna Bacon, Esmita Charani, Jane Turton, Rebecca Guy, Samuel Lipworth, Aleksandra Borek, Simon Collin, Diane Ashiru-Oredope, Gisela Robles Aguilar, Nichola Naylor, Alice Ledda, Ross Booton, Amelia Andrews, Mark Sutton, Ginny Moore, Nicole Stoesser, Donna Lecky, Hannah Higgins, Caroline Jamieson-Leadbitter, Sarah Tonkin-Crine, Alison Holmes, and Sarah A Walker. The authors would also like to acknowledge the ESPAUR oversight group members.

Conflicts of Interest: The authors declare no conflict of interest.

References

1. Ashiru-Oredope, D.; Hopkins, S. on behalf of the English Surveillance Programme for Antimicrobial Utilization and Resistance Oversight Group; Kessel, A.; Hopkins, S.; Ashiru-Oredope, D.; Brown, B.; Brown, N.; Carter, S.; Charlett, A.; Cichowka, A.; et al. Antimicrobial stewardship: English surveillance programme for antimicrobial utilization and resistance (ESPAUR). *J. Antimicrob. Chemother.* **2013**, *68*, 2421–2423. [CrossRef] [PubMed]
2. Agnew, E.; Robotham, J. on behalf of the ESPAUR Research Chapter Authors. Chapter 8. Research. In *English Surveillance Programme for Antimicrobial Utilisation and Resistance (ESPAUR) Report 2021 to 2022*; UK Health Security Agency: London, UK, 2022.
3. *UK 5-Year Action Plan for Antimicrobial Resistance 2019 to 2024*; Department of Health and Social Care: London, UK, 2019.
4. Acolatse, J.E.E.; Portal, E.A.R.; Boostrom, I.; Akafity, G.; Dakroah, M.P.; Chalker, V.J.; Sands, K.; Spiller, O.B. Environmental surveillance of ESBL and carbapenemase-producing gram-negative bacteria in a Ghanaian Tertiary Hospital. *Antimicrob. Resist. Infect. Control.* **2022**, *11*, 1–15. [CrossRef] [PubMed]
5. Aliabadi, S.; Jauneikaite, E.; Müller-Pebody, B.; Hope, R.; Vihta, K.-D.; Horner, C.; Costelloe, C.E. Exploring temporal trends and risk factors for resistance in *Escherichia coli*-causing bacteraemia in England between 2013 and 2018: An ecological study. *J. Antimicrob. Chemother.* **2022**, *77*, 782–792. [CrossRef] [PubMed]
6. Allen, H.; Merrick, R.; Ivanov, Z.; Pitt, R.; Mohammed, H.; Sinka, K.; Hughes, G.; Fifer, H.; Cole, M.J. Is there an association between previous infection with *Neisseria gonorrhoeae* and gonococcal AMR? A cross-sectional analysis of national and sentinel surveillance data in England, 2015–2019. *Sex. Transm. Infect.* **2023**, *99*, 1–6. [CrossRef] [PubMed]
7. Andrews, A.; Bou-Antoun, S.; Guy, R.; Brown, C.S.; Hopkins, S.; Gerver, S. Respiratory antibacterial prescribing in primary care and the COVID-19 pandemic in England, winter season 2020–21. *J. Antimicrob. Chemother.* **2021**, *77*, 799–802. [CrossRef] [PubMed]
8. Andrews, A.; Budd, E.L.; Hendrick, A.; Ashiru-Oredope, D.; Beech, E.; Hopkins, S.; Gerver, S.; Muller-Pebody, B.; The Amu Covid-Stakeholder Group. Surveillance of antibacterial usage during the COVID-19 pandemic in England, 2020. *Antibiotics* **2021**, *10*, 841. [CrossRef] [PubMed]
9. Aranega-Bou, P.; Ellaby, N.; Ellington, M.J.; Moore, G. Migration of Escherichia coli and Klebsiella pneumoniae Carbapenemase (KPC)-Producing Enterobacter cloacae through wastewater pipework and establishment in hospital sink waste traps in a laboratory model system. *Microorganisms* **2021**, *9*, 1868. [CrossRef]
10. Baede, V.O.; David, M.Z.; Andrasevic, A.T.; Blanc, D.S.; Borg, M.; Brennan, G.; Catry, B.; Chabaud, A.; Empel, J.; Enger, H.; et al. MRSA surveillance programmes worldwide: Moving towards a harmonised international approach. *Int. J. Antimicrob. Agents* **2022**, *59*, 106538. [CrossRef]

11. Beale, M.A.; Marks, M.; Cole, M.J.; Lee, M.K.; Pitt, R.; Ruis, C.; Balla, E.; Crucitti, T.; Ewens, M.; Fernández-Naval, C.; et al. Global phylogeny of Treponema pallidum lineages reveals recent expansion and spread of contemporary syphilis. *Nat. Microbiol.* **2021**, *6*, 1549–1560. [CrossRef]
12. Berrocal-Almanza, L.C.; Harris, R.J.; Collin, S.M.; Muzyamba, M.C.; Conroy, O.D.; Mirza, A.; O'Connell, A.M.; Altass, L. Anderson, S.R.; Thomas, H.L.; et al. Effectiveness of nationwide programmatic testing and treatment for latent tuberculosis infection in migrants in England: A retrospective, population-based cohort study. *Lancet Public Health* **2022**, *7*, e305–e315. [CrossRef]
13. Bhate, K.; Lin, L.Y.; Barbieri, J.; Leyrat, C.; Hopkins, S.; Stabler, R.; Shallcross, L.; Smeeth, L.; Francis, N.A.; Mathur, R.; et al. Is there an association between long-term antibiotics for acne and subsequent infection sequelae and antimicrobial resistance? A systematic review protocol. *BMJ Open* **2020**, *10*, e033662. [CrossRef] [PubMed]
14. Bhattacharya, A.; Collin, S.M.; Stimson, J.; Thelwall, S.; Nsonwu, O.; Gerver, S.; Robotham, J.; Wilcox, M.; Hopkins, S.; Hope, R. Healthcare-associated COVID-19 in England: A national data linkage study. *J. Infect.* **2021**, *83*, 565–572. [CrossRef] [PubMed]
15. Bielicki, J.A.; Stöhr, W.; Barratt, S.; Dunn, D.; Naufal, N.; Roland, D.; Sturgeon, K.; Finn, A.; Rodriguez-Ruiz, J.P.; Malhotra-Kumar, S.; et al. Effect of amoxicillin dose and treatment duration on the need for antibiotic Re-treatment in children with community-acquired pneumonia: The CAP-IT randomized clinical trial. *JAMA* **2021**, *326*, 1713–1724. [CrossRef] [PubMed]
16. Borek, A.J.; Pouwels, K.B.; van Hecke, O.; Robotham, J.V.; Butler, C.C.; Tonkin-Crine, S. Role of locum GPs in antibiotic prescribing and stewardship: A mixed-methods study. *Br. J. Gen. Pract.* **2022**, *72*, e118–e127. [CrossRef]
17. Buchanan, J.; Roope, L.S.J.; Morrell, L.; Pouwels, K.B.; Robotham, J.V.; Abel, L.; Crook, D.W.; Peto, T.; Butler, C.C.; Walker, A.S.; et al. Preferences for medical consultations from online providers: Evidence from a discrete choice experiment in the United Kingdom. *Appl. Health Econ. Health Policy* **2021**, *19*, 521–535. [CrossRef] [PubMed]
18. Budgell, E.P.; Davies, T.J.; Donker, T.; Hopkins, S.; Wyllie, D.H.; Peto, T.E.A.; Gill, M.J.; Llewelyn, M.J.; Walker, A.S. Impact of antibiotic use on patient-level risk of death in 36 million hospital admissions in England. *J. Infect.* **2022**, *84*, 311–320. [CrossRef] [PubMed]
19. Coia, J.E.; Wilson, J.A.; Bak, A.; Marsden, G.L.; Shimonovich, M.; Loveday, H.P.; Humphreys, H.; Wigglesworth, N.; Demirjian, A.; Brooks, J.; et al. Joint Healthcare Infection Society (HIS) and Infection Prevention Society (IPS) guidelines for the prevention and control of meticillin-resistant *Staphylococcus aureus* (MRSA) in healthcare facilities. *J. Hosp. Infect.* **2021**, *118*, S1–S39. [CrossRef]
20. Cole, M.J.; Davis, G.S.; Fifer, H.; Saunders, J.M.; Unemo, M.; Hadad, R.; Roberts, D.J.; Fazal, M.; Day, M.J.; Minshul, J.; et al. No widespread dissemination of Chlamydia trachomatis diagnostic-escape variants and the impact of *Neisseria gonorrhoeae* positivity on the Aptima Combo 2 assay. *Sex. Transm. Infect.* **2022**, *98*, 366–370. [CrossRef]
21. Collin, S.M.; Farra, A. Antimicrobial resistance, infection prevention and control, and conflict in the Middle East. *Int. J. Infect. Dis.* **2021**, *111*, 326–327. [CrossRef]
22. Dean, G.; Soni, S.; Pitt, R.; Ross, J.; Sabin, C.; Whetham, J. Treatment of mild-to-moderate pelvic inflammatory disease with a short-course azithromycin-based regimen versus ofloxacin plus metronidazole: Results of a multicentre, randomised controlled trial. *Sex. Transm. Infect.* **2021**, *97*, 177–182. [CrossRef]
23. Emes, D.; Naylor, N.; Waage, J.; Knight, G. Quantifying the relationship between antibiotic use in food-producing animals and antibiotic resistance in humans. *Antibiotics* **2022**, *11*, 66. [CrossRef]
24. Fifer, H.; Livermore, D.M.; Uthayakumaran, T.; Woodford, N.; Cole, M.J. What's left in the cupboard? Older antimicrobials for treating gonorrhoea. *J. Antimicrob. Chemother.* **2021**, *76*, 1215–1220. [CrossRef] [PubMed]
25. Fifer, H.; Merrick, R.; Pitt, R.; Yung, M.; Allen, H.; Day, M.; Sinka, K.; Woodford, N.; Mohammed, H.; Brown, C.S.; et al. Frequency and correlates of *Mycoplasma genitalium* antimicrobial resistance mutations and their association with treatment outcomes: Findings from a national sentinel surveillance pilot in England. *Sex. Transm. Dis.* **2021**, *48*, 951–954. [CrossRef] [PubMed]
26. Fifer, H.; Schaefer, U.; Pitt, R.; Allen, H.; Day, M.; Woodford, N.; Cole, M.J. Use of genomics to investigate *Neisseria gonorrhoeae* antimicrobial susceptibility testing discrepancies. *J. Antimicrob. Chemother.* **2022**, *77*, 849–850. [CrossRef] [PubMed]
27. Gagliotti, C.; Högberg, L.D.; Billström, H.; Eckmanns, T.; Giske, C.G.; Heuer, O.E.; Jarlier, V.; Kahlmeter, G.; Lo Fo Wong, D.; Monen, J.; et al. *Staphylococcus aureus* bloodstream infections: Diverging trends of meticillin-resistant and meticillin-susceptible isolates, EU/EEA, 2005 to 2018. *Eurosurveillance* **2021**, *26*, 2002094. [CrossRef] [PubMed]
28. Gerver, S.M.; Nsonwu, O.; Thelwall, S.; Brown, C.S.; Hope, R. Trends in rates of incidence, fatality and antimicrobial resistance among isolates of *Pseudomonas* spp. causing bloodstream infections in England between 2009 and 2018: Results from a national voluntary surveillance scheme. *J. Hosp. Infect.* **2022**, *120*, 73–80. [CrossRef]
29. Hayes, C.V.; Eley, C.V.; Ashiru-Oredope, D.; Hann, M.; McNulty, C.A. Development and pilot evaluation of an educational programme on infection prevention and antibiotics with English and Scottish youth groups, informed by COM-B. *J. Infect. Prev.* **2021**, *22*, 212–219. [CrossRef]
30. Hayes, C.V.; Eley, C.V.; Wood, F.; Demirjian, A.; McNulty, C.A.M. Knowledge and attitudes of adolescents towards the human microbiome and antibiotic resistance: A qualitative study. *JAC-Antimicrob. Resist.* **2021**, *3*, dlab039. [CrossRef]
31. Hayes, C.V.; Mahon, B.; Sides, E.; Allison, R.; Lecky, D.M.; McNulty, C.A.M. Empowering patients to self-manage common infections: Qualitative study informing the development of an evidence-based patient information leaflet. *Antibiotics* **2021**, *10*, 1113. [CrossRef]
32. Horner, C.; Mushtaq, S.; Allen, M.; Hope, R.; Gerver, S.; Longshaw, C.; Reynolds, R.; Woodford, N.; Livermore, D.M. Replacement of *Enterococcus faecalis* by *Enterococcus faecium* as the predominant enterococcus in UK bacteraemias. *JAC-Antimicrob. Resist.* **2021**, *3*, dlab185. [CrossRef]

33. Khan, U.B.; Jauneikaite, E.; Andrews, R.; Chalker, V.J.; Spiller, O.B. Identifying large-scale recombination and capsular switching events in *Streptococcus agalactiae* strains causing disease in adults in the UK between 2014 and 2015. *Microb. Genom.* **2022**, *8*, 000783. [CrossRef] [PubMed]
34. Lamagni, T.; Wloch, C.; Broughton, K.; Collin, S.M.; Chalker, V.; Coelho, J.; Ladhani, S.N.; Brown, C.S.; Shetty, N.; Johnson, A.P. Assessing the added value of group B Streptococcus maternal immunisation in preventing maternal infection and fetal harm: Population surveillance study. *BJOG* **2022**, *129*, 233–240. [CrossRef] [PubMed]
35. Langton Hewer, S.C.; Smyth, A.R.; Brown, M.; Jones, A.P.; Hickey, H.; Kenna, D.; Ashby, D.; Thompson, A.; Sutton, L.; Clayton, D.; et al. Intravenous or oral antibiotic treatment in adults and children with cystic fibrosis and Pseudomonas aeruginosa infection: The TORPEDO-CF RCT. *Health Technol. Assess.* **2021**, *25*, 1–128. [CrossRef] [PubMed]
36. Larsen, J.; Raisen, C.L.; Ba, X.L.; Sadgrove, N.J.; Padilla-González, G.F.; Simmonds, M.S.J.; Loncaric, I.; Kerschner, H.; Apfalter, P.; Hartl, R.; et al. Emergence of methicillin resistance predates the clinical use of antibiotics. *Nature* **2022**, *602*, 135–141. [CrossRef] [PubMed]
37. Lipworth, S.; Vihta, K.-D.; Chau, K.; Barker, L.; George, S.; Kavanagh, J.; Davies, T.; Vaughan, A.; Andersson, M.; Jeffery, K.; et al. Ten-year longitudinal molecular epidemiology study of *Escherichia coli* and *Klebsiella* species bloodstream infections in Oxfordshire, UK. *Genome Med.* **2021**, *13*, 1–13. [CrossRef] [PubMed]
38. Lopez-Diaz, M.; Ellaby, N.; Turton, J.; Woodford, N.; Tomas, M.; Ellington, M.J. NDM-1 carbapenemase resistance gene vehicles emergent on distinct plasmid backbones from the IncL/M family. *J. Antimicrob. Chemother.* **2022**, *77*, 620–624. [CrossRef] [PubMed]
39. Mabayoje, D.A.; Kenna, D.T.D.; Dance, D.A.B.; NicFhogartaigh, C. Melioidosis manifesting as chronic femoral osteomyelitis in patient from Ghana. *Emerg. Infect. Dis.* **2022**, *28*, 201–204. [CrossRef]
40. Martelli, F.; AbuOun, M.; Cawthraw, S.; Storey, N.; Turner, O.; Ellington, M.; Nair, S.; Painset, A.; Teale, C.; Anjum, M.F. Detection of the transferable tigecycline resistance gene tet (X4) in *Escherichia coli* from pigs in the United Kingdom. *J. Antimicrob. Chemother.* **2022**, *77*, 846–848. [CrossRef]
41. McHardy, J.A.; Selvaganeshapillai, V.; Khanna, P.; Whittington, A.M.; Turton, J.; Gopal Rao, G. A case of neck abscess caused by rare hypervirulent *Klebsiella pneumoniae*, capsular type K20 and sequence type 420. *Ann. Clin. Microbiol. Antimicrob.* **2021**, *20*, 46. [CrossRef]
42. McHugh, M.P.; Parcell, B.J.; Pettigrew, K.A.; Toner, G.; Khatamzas, E.; El Sakka, N.; Karcher, A.M.; Walker, J.; Weir, R.; Meunier, D.; et al. Presence of optrA-mediated linezolid resistance in multiple lineages and plasmids of *Enterococcus faecalis* revealed by long read sequencing. *Microbiology* **2022**, *168*, 001137. [CrossRef]
43. McNulty, C.; Read, B.; Quigley, A.; Verlander, N.Q.; Lecky, D.M. What the public in England know about antibiotic use and resistance in 2020: A face-to-face questionnaire survey. *BMJ Open* **2022**, *12*, e055464. [CrossRef] [PubMed]
44. McNulty, C.; Sides, E.; Thomas, A.; Kamal, A.; Syeda, R.B.; Kaissi, A.; Lecky, D.M.; Patel, M.; Campos-Matos, I.; Shukla, R.; et al. Public views of and reactions to the COVID-19 pandemic in England-a qualitative study with diverse ethnicities. *BMJ Open* **2022**, *12*, e061027. [CrossRef] [PubMed]
45. Meunier, D.; Woodford, N.; Hopkins, K.L. Evaluation of the Revogene Carba C assay for detection of carbapenemases in MDR Gram-negative bacteria. *J. Antimicrob. Chemother.* **2021**, *76*, 1941–1944. [CrossRef]
46. Moore, A.; Cannings-John, R.; Butler, C.C.; McNulty, C.A.; Francis, N.A. Alternative approaches to managing respiratory tract infections: A survey of public perceptions. *BJGP Open* **2021**, *5*, 1–12. [CrossRef] [PubMed]
47. Morrell, L.; Buchanan, J.; Roope, L.S.J.; Pouwels, K.B.; Butler, C.C.; Hayhoe, B.; Tonkin-Crine, S.; McLeod, M.; Robotham, J.V.; Holmes, A.; et al. Public preferences for delayed or immediate antibiotic prescriptions in UK primary care: A choice experiment. *PLoS Med.* **2021**, *18*, e1003737. [CrossRef]
48. Muller-Pebody, B.; Sinnathamby, M.A.; Warburton, F.; Rooney, G.; Andrews, N.; Whitaker, H.; Henderson, K.L.; Tsang, C.; Hopkins, S.; Pebody, R.G.; et al. Impact of the childhood influenza vaccine programme on antibiotic prescribing rates in primary care in England. *Vaccine* **2021**, *39*, 6622–6627. [CrossRef]
49. Murray, C.J.; Ikuta, K.S.; Sharara, F.; Swetschinski, L.; Aguilar, G.R.; Gray, A.; Han, C.; Bisignano, C.; Rao, P.; Wool, E.; et al. Global burden of bacterial antimicrobial resistance in 2019: A systematic analysis. *Lancet* **2022**, *399*, 629–655. [CrossRef]
50. Patel, S.; Jhass, A.; Slee, A.; Hopkins, S.; Shallcross, L. Variation in approaches to antimicrobial use surveillance in high-income secondary care settings: A systematic review. *J. Antimicrob. Chemother.* **2021**, *76*, 1969–1977. [CrossRef]
51. Pitt, R.; Fifer, H.; Woodford, N.; Hopkins, S.; Cole, M.J. Prevalence of *Chlamydia trachomatis* and *Mycoplasma genitalium* coinfections and *M. genitalium* antimicrobial resistance in rectal specimens. *Sex. Transm. Infect.* **2021**, *97*, 469–470. [CrossRef]
52. Sánchez-Busó, L.; Yeats, C.A.; Taylor, B.; Goater, R.J.; Underwood, A.; Abudahab, K.; Argimón, S.; Ma, K.C.; Mortimer, T.D.; Golparian, D.; et al. A community-driven resource for genomic epidemiology and antimicrobial resistance prediction of *Neisseria gonorrhoeae* at Pathogenwatch. *Genome Med.* **2021**, *13*, 61. [CrossRef]
53. Sides, E.; Jones, L.F.; Kamal, A.; Thomas, A.; Syeda, R., Kaissi, A.; Lecky, D.M.; Patel, M.; Nellums, L.; Greenway, J.; et al. Attitudes towards coronavirus (COVID-19) vaccine and sources of information across diverse ethnic groups in the UK: A qualitative study from June to October 2020. *BMJ Open* **2022**, *12*, e060992. [CrossRef] [PubMed]
54. Sloot, R.; Nsonwu, O.; Chudasama, D.; Rooney, G.; Pearson, C.; Choi, H.; Mason, E.; Springer, A.; Gerver, S.; Brown, C.; et al. Rising rates of hospital-onset *Klebsiella* spp. and *Pseudomonas aeruginosa* bacteraemia in NHS acute trusts in England: A review of national surveillance data, August 2020–February 2021. *J. Hosp. Infect.* **2022**, *119*, 175–181. [CrossRef] [PubMed]

55. Syeda, R.; Touboul Lundgren, P.; Kasza, G.; Truninger, M.; Brown, C.; Lacroix-Hugues, V.; Izsó, T.; Teixeira, P.; Eley, C.; Ferré, N.; et al. Young People's Views on Food Hygiene and Food Safety: A Multicentre Qualitative Study. *Educ. Sci.* **2021**, *11*, 261. [CrossRef]
56. Taylor, E.; Bal, A.M.; Balakrishnan, I.; Brown, N.M.; Burns, P.; Clark, M.; Diggle, M.; Donaldson, H.; Eltringham, I.; Folb, J.; et al. A prospective surveillance study to determine the prevalence of 16S rRNA methyltransferase-producing Gram-negative bacteria in the UK. *J. Antimicrob. Chemother.* **2021**, *76*, 2428–2436. [CrossRef] [PubMed]
57. Taylor, E.; Jauneikaite, E.; Sriskandan, S.; Woodford, N.; Hopkins, K.L. Detection and characterisation of 16S rRNA methyltransferase-producing *Pseudomonas aeruginosa* from the UK and Republic of Ireland from 2003–2015. *Int. J. Antimicrob. Agents* **2022**, *59*, 106550. [CrossRef] [PubMed]
58. Unemo, M.; Ahlstrand, J.; Sánchez-Busó, L.; Day, M.; Aanensen, D.; Golparian, D.; Jacobsson, S.; Cole, M.J.; European Collaborative Group. High susceptibility to zoliflodacin and conserved target (GyrB) for zoliflodacin among 1209 consecutive clinical *Neisseria gonorrhoeae* isolates from 25 European countries, 2018. *J. Antimicrob. Chemother.* **2021**, *76*, 1221–1228. [CrossRef] [PubMed]
59. Unemo, M.; Lahra, M.M.; Escher, M.; Eremin, S.; Cole, M.J.; Galarza, P.; Ndowa, F.; Martin, I.; Dillon, J.R.; Galas, M.; et al. WHO global antimicrobial resistance surveillance for *Neisseria gonorrhoeae* 2017–18: A retrospective observational study. *Lancet Microbe.* **2021**, *2*, e627–e636. [CrossRef]
60. Zendri, F.; Isgren, C.M.; Sinovich, M.; Richards-Rios, P.; Hopkins, K.L.; Russell, K.; Groves, N.; Litt, D.; Fry, N.K.; Timofte, D. Case report: Toxigenic *Corynebacterium ulcerans* diphtheria-like infection in a horse in the United Kingdom. *Front. Vet. Sci.* **2021**, *8*, 650238. [CrossRef]
61. Zhu, N.J.; Ahmad, R.; Holmes, A.; Robotham, J.V.; Lebcir, R.; Atun, R. System dynamics modelling to formulate policy interventions to optimise antibiotic prescribing in hospitals. *J. Oper. Res. Soc.* **2020**, *72*, 2490–2502. [CrossRef]

Disclaimer/Publisher's Note: The statements, opinions and data contained in all publications are solely those of the individual author(s) and contributor(s) and not of MDPI and/or the editor(s). MDPI and/or the editor(s) disclaim responsibility for any injury to people or property resulting from any ideas, methods, instructions or products referred to in the content.

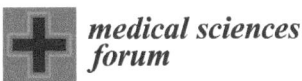

Proceeding Paper

Farm Vet Champion Delivery of Training and SMART Goal Setting to Improve Antimicrobial Stewardship in Farm Veterinary Practice [†]

Fiona Lovatt *, Lucy Coyne, Amy Thompson, Georgia Monaghan, Ashley Doorly and Chris Gush

RCVS Knowledge, The Cursitor, 38 Chancery Lane, London WC2A 1EN, UK

* Correspondence: fiona@rcvsknowledge.org; Tel.: +44-(0)20-7202-0721
† Presented at the 6th Antibiotic Guardian Shared Learning and Awards, Antibiotic Guardian, 2 May 2023; Available online: https://antibioticguardian.com/antibiotic-guardian-2022-shared-learning-awards/.

Abstract: Farm Vet Champions (FVC) is a collaborative project to unite and empower UK farm vets to establish, embed, and champion responsible antimicrobial stewardship. FVCs support the veterinary profession to improve animal health and welfare standards and provide positive inspiration and leadership towards One Health efforts. The initiative provides farm vets and their teams with free online learning, and an online tool that encourages users to set goals that are specific, measurable, achievable, and realistic, within a set time limit.

Keywords: antimicrobial stewardship; veterinary; livestock; education; SMART goal

1. Project Overview

Farm Vet Champions (FVC) is a collaborative project to unite and empower UK farm vets to establish, embed, and champion responsible antimicrobial stewardship. FVCs support the veterinary profession to continue to improve animal health and welfare standards and provide positive inspiration and leadership towards One Health efforts.

Farm Vet Champions online learning is accessible for free to all veterinary practice team members and offers bite-sized learning, with users able to select the format (webinars, podcasts) and topics that are most relevant to them. The FVC mantra is to plan, prevent, and protect herds and flocks by predicting disease threats and reviewing animal husbandry and environmental influences on livestock health. FVC also provides users with a SMART goals tool that supports the sustained translation of learning into practice and can be set at an individual or team level. SMART goals are specific, measurable, attainable, realistic, and time-bound goals that help teams turn learning into action.

FVC is led by RCVS Knowledge (London, UK) [1], the charity partner of the Royal College of Veterinary Surgeons (RCVS), an impartial organisation that collaborates with veterinary stakeholders to provide evidence-based educational materials and promote quality improvement in veterinary practice. RCVS Knowledge is driving behaviour changes in responsible antimicrobial use by improving access to responsible antimicrobial use knowledge for UK farm veterinary practice teams and helping teams to apply their learning to demonstrate accountability and monitor achievements.

As part of Farm Vet Champions, RCVS Knowledge has established an ambassador group of motivated UK farm vets committed to championing responsible antimicrobial use and sharing knowledge. Through education, the SMART goals tool, and the ambassador network, FVC highlights the importance of collaboration in the success of this mission; collaboration that is cultivated both in the practice setting and out on farms with farmers and clients.

2. Outcomes and Impact

By December 2022, 800 people had signed up to access the Farm Vet Champion platform. Of these, 500 were RCVS-registered veterinary professionals prepared to pledge commitment to driving antimicrobial stewardship forward in practice and on farms. RCVS registrations suggest there are 3315 farm vets in the UK.

FVC has brought major UK veterinary organisations together, collaborating to drive the core message, 'Plan, Prevent Protect'. Over 41 organisations are part of the Farm Vet Champions stakeholder group, and all UK livestock veterinary associations contribute to the steering group, which has included providing learning materials.

Case study examples have shown effective implementation of 'Plan Prevent Protect'. In one example [2] a farm client was experiencing a daily mortality rate of 1% due to multi-drug resistant E. coli associated egg peritonitis. An on-farm investigation by a FVC revealed a series of health, welfare, and management issues.

Working with the farmer, a plan was made to improve flock health, which incorporated the use of vaccinations, vaccination auditing, improved farm biosecurity and water hygiene, parasite monitoring and control, and environmental management and enrichment. In the next flock cycle, the farm saw over 50% increase in net profit compared to the previous flock. The flock's egg production and other production parameters remained above target for the entirety of the flock's production cycle, demonstrating the improvement in health and welfare that had been achieved through the interventions.

Through planning and consideration around prevention techniques, the flock was protected. This is just one example of how putting the FVC principles of 'Plan Prevent Protect' into action can influence the industry and reduce the use of antibiotics.

3. Future Development

The Farm Vet Champions' ambition is to make a difference in every veterinary practice, at the point of every vet-farmer conversation. RCVS Knowledge will continue to work with the FVC ambassador group of forward-thinking individuals, in order to widen its reach within the veterinary community. The aim is to establish inclusive and sustainable FVC communities on local, regional, and virtual levels. These groups will share ideas, set and track SMART goals to monitor progress, and showcase good practices for implementation.

The production of "in conversation with ... " podcasts [3] will continue to allow topical focus on more specific subjects (such as the challenges faced in the lambing season or the 'Plan Prevent Protect' application to backyard hens).

There is an ongoing commitment to promote and recruit new Farm Vet Champions, with a focus around students and recently qualified vets, in order to empower the next generation of farm vets in championing responsible antimicrobial use for the benefit of vets, clients, farmers, animals, and society.

Author Contributions: Conceptualization, F.L., A.D. and C.G.; methodology: F.L., L.C., A.T., A.D. and C.G.; writing–original draft preparation: F.L., L.C., A.T., G.M. and A.D.; writing–review and editing: F.L., A.D. and C.G.; project administration: L.C., A.T. and G.M.; funding acquisition: F.L., A.D. and C.G. All authors have read and agreed to the published version of the manuscript.

Funding: The initial project was funded by the Veterinary Medicines Directorate (VMD).

Institutional Review Board Statement: Not applicable.

Informed Consent Statement: Not applicable.

Data Availability Statement: All data generated as a result of the work outlined are unavailable due to privacy reasons.

Acknowledgments: With thanks to Alex Royden, who submitted her FVC case study.

Conflicts of Interest: The authors declare no conflict of interest.

References

1. RCVS Knowledge. Available online: https://rcvsknowledge.org.uk/amr (accessed on 16 December 2022).
2. Alex Royden Reduction of Antimicrobial Use on Layer Site AMR FVC. Available online: https://knowledge.rcvs.org.uk/document-library/reduction-of-antimicrobial-use-on-layer-site/ (accessed on 13 February 2022).
3. Farm Vet Champions. Available online: https://rcvsknowledge.podbean.com/category/farm-vet-champions (accessed on 13 February 2022).

Disclaimer/Publisher's Note: The statements, opinions and data contained in all publications are solely those of the individual author(s) and contributor(s) and not of MDPI and/or the editor(s). MDPI and/or the editor(s) disclaim responsibility for any injury to people or property resulting from any ideas, methods, instructions or products referred to in the content.

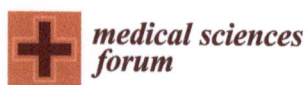

Proceeding Paper

Supporting Timely IV to Oral Antibiotic Switch through Development of Accessible Clinical Decision Tools [†]

Balwinder Bolla [1,*], Tom Rennison [2], Catherine Cox [2], Rupen Tamang [2], Magda Krupczak [1] and Yui Ka Ho [1]

[1] Department of Pharmacy, United Lincolnshire Hospitals NHS Trust, Lincoln County Hospital, Lincoln LN25QY, UK
[2] Post Graduate Medical Education Centre (PGMEC), United Lincolnshire Hospitals NHS Trust, Lincoln County Hospital, Lincoln LN25QY, UK
* Correspondence: balwinder.bolla@ulh.nhs.uk; Tel.: +44-(0)15-2257-3715
[†] Presented at the 6th Antibiotic Guardian Shared Learning and Awards, Antibiotic Guardian, 2 May 2023; Available online: https://antibioticguardian.com/antibiotic-guardian-2022-shared-learning-awards/.

Abstract: The timely and appropriate IV to Oral Switch (IVOS) of antibiotics is beneficial to patient care and AMR strategies. However, a lack of prescriber confidence in deciding to switch often prolongs IV antibiotic use. The creation of a bite-size educational video and a smartphone application clinical decision tool, has brought the learning process closer to everyday practice, in an easy to access and understandable manner. Both have been very well received and shared with many acute NHS Trusts. The implementation was correlated with an improvement in audit findings. The multidisciplinary and collaborative approach in developing these tools has been the key to success.

Keywords: antibiotic; antimicrobial; intravenous; clinical decision tool; IVOS; oral switch

1. Project Overview

The IV to Oral Switch (IVOS) of antibiotics is often unnecessarily delayed due to lack of confidence and knowledge around when it is appropriate to initiate it. This impacts antimicrobial resistance, patient outcomes, bed flow in hospitals, and the utilisation of nursing skill in acute NHS Trusts. Junior doctors are usually tasked with IVOS but are hesitant to push or challenge the hierarchy in clinical teams towards this, without robust support. This is also fuelled by senior decision makers being critical of whether sufficient rationale and logic have been applied. This lends to a 'just-in-case' approach of continuing IV antibiotics for longer than needed.

The parameters to apply for safe and effective IVOS are covered in antibiotic policy and guidelines within United Lincolnshire Hospitals Trust, but these are not easy to access or recall in daily practice, causing this aspect of stewardship to be difficult to implement [1].

A redesign of IVOS snapshot audits undertaken in the Trust revealed that use of IV antibiotics was appropriate in 84% of the audited cases. More interestingly, the auditors (a mix of doctors, nurses, and pharmacists) provided positive feedback on the educational and interventional value of the new audit tool, even for non-prescribers, due to the logical order in which questions were presented and the specifying of parameters on the form itself.

The feedback from this audit highlighted the potential to raise awareness, knowledge, and application of IVOS, in a way that is more accessible and easy to absorb in clinical practice.

2. Outcomes and Impact

The PGMEC's success with publishing antibiotic teaching sessions to their ULHT YouTube channel during the pandemic, prompted creation of a video on IVOS. This video presents the questions, explanation, and logical order of the audit form, which allows for direct application to clinical cases by staff. The video was sent out in various communications

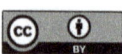

across the Trust to all staff groups, with additional direct PGMEC emails to all prescribers and pharmacists. For further accessibility, a QR code linked to the video was added to mandatory antibiotic posters, displayed on all clinical areas throughout the Trust.

To further enhance the accessibility and application of IVOS considerations at the patient bedside, a clinical decision tool was developed for use via the smartphone app MicroGuide ®(Induction Healthcare Group PLC, London, UK). Despite some limitations on how the information is presented, tests confirmed the validity of output.

The positive qualitative feedback received from a wide variety of staff members and their perspectives included: highly educational, easy to use, clear, and concise. The ability to support nurses' competency levels, improve documentation, and ease workforce pressure via confident clinical decisions has potential to improve bed flow through hospitals. Both the tool and video have been shared regionally and nationally, with over 30 acute NHS Trusts.

The audit data on the appropriateness of IV antibiotic prescriptions over 72 hours showed an improvement to 100% (Table S1). This was following an intense awareness campaign with the IVOS video and launch of the MicroGuide ®IVOS clinical decision tool, alongside direct presentations to multidisciplinary staff of all levels.

3. Future Development

The tool will be further developed based on feedback. Plans are underway to explore the incorporation of our tool into patient's medical notes once digitalisation occurs at ULHT. Regular awareness campaigns will be needed to tie in with junior doctor's annual changeovers and to capture new members of staff, including agency staff. This should cover multidisciplinary support, with junior and senior medical and nursing staff, bed managers, and non-clinical colleagues keen to utilise the tools for confident, prompt, and timely decisions. The collaborative approach to the promotion and utilisation of these tools has and will be the key to success.

Using audit or surveillance to capture the effect on the reduction in the consumption of broad-spectrum antimicrobials, reduction in IV line infections, reduction in the length of antibiotic course, and reduction in the length of stay in hospital would be a challenge, but would also be valuable if accomplished. Such insight would further drive support to embed IVOS into prescribing practice.

Supplementary Materials: The following supporting information can be downloaded at: https://www.mdpi.com/article/10.3390/msf2022015006/s1.

Author Contributions: Conceptualization, B.B.; methodology, B.B.; software, T.R. and M.K.; validation, M.K. and Y.K.H.; formal analysis, B.B. and C.C.; resources, R.T., T.R. and C.C.; data curation, B.B. and T.R.; writing—original draft preparation, B.B.; writing—review and editing, B.B. and R.T.; visualization, B.B.; supervision, B.B.; project administration, M.K. All authors have read and agreed to the published version of the manuscript.

Funding: This research received no external funding.

Institutional Review Board Statement: Not applicable.

Informed Consent Statement: Not applicable.

Data Availability Statement: The data presented in this study are available in Figure S1 and Table S1.

Acknowledgments: The authors would like to thank Induction Healthcare Group PLC (Guidance-Induction Healthcare Group), for developing the MicroGuide ®platform which enabled development of this clinical decision tool.

Conflicts of Interest: The authors declare no conflict of interest.

Reference

1. Antimicrobial Intravenous-to-oral Switch: Criteria for Early Switch. Available online: https://www.gov.uk/government/publications/antimicrobial-intravenous-to-oral-switch-criteria-for-early-switch (accessed on 16 December 2022).

Disclaimer/Publisher's Note: The statements, opinions and data contained in all publications are solely those of the individual author(s) and contributor(s) and not of MDPI and/or the editor(s). MDPI and/or the editor(s) disclaim responsibility for any injury to people or property resulting from any ideas, methods, instructions or products referred to in the content.

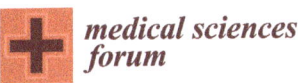

Proceeding Paper

Scaling-Up Interventions for Strengthening Antimicrobial Stewardship Using a One Health Approach in Wakiso District, Uganda †

Grace Biyinzika Lubega [1,*], David Musoke [1], Suzan Nakalawa [1], Claire Brandish [2], Bee Yean Ng [3], Filimin Niyongabo [1], Freddy Eric Kitutu [4], Jagdeep Gheer [2], Jody Winter [5], Michael Obeng Brown [6], Kate Russell-Hobbs [2], Lawrence Mugisha [7] and Linda Gibson [6]

1. Department of Disease Control and Environmental Health, School of Public Health, College of Health Sciences, Makerere University, Kampala P.O. Box 7072, Uganda
2. Pharmacy Department, Buckinghamshire Healthcare NHS Trust, Aylesbury HP21 8AL, UK
3. Department of Pharmacy, Oxford University Hospitals NHS Foundation Trust, Oxford OX3 9DU, UK
4. Department of Pharmacy, School of Health Sciences, College of Health Sciences, Makerere University, Kampala P.O. Box 7072, Uganda
5. Department of Biosciences, School of Science and Technology, Nottingham Trent University, Nottingham NG11 8NS, UK
6. Institute of Health and Allied Professions, School of Social Sciences, Nottingham Trent University, Nottingham NG1 4FQ, UK
7. Department for Livestock and Industrial Resources, School of Veterinary Medicine and Animal Resources, College of Veterinary Medicine, Animal Resources and Bio-security, Makerere University, Kampala P.O. Box 7062, Uganda

* Correspondence: glubega@musph.ac.ug
† Presented at the 6th Antibiotic Guardian Shared Learning and Awards, Antibiotic Guardian, 2 May 2023; Available online: https://antibioticguardian.com/antibiotic-guardian-2022-shared-learning-awards/.

Abstract: We implemented a multidisciplinary project between Uganda and the UK aimed at strengthening antimicrobial stewardship (AMS) in Wakiso district, with a focus on capacity building, stakeholder engagement, and knowledge exchange using a One Health approach. Project activities included: trainings and workshops on antimicrobial resistance (AMR), AMS, infection prevention and control (IPC); Global Point Prevalence Survey (GPPS) data collection and analysis; and the mentorship of lower level health facilities. Our project demonstrated that AMS interventions using a One Health approach can enhance understanding of the prudent use of antimicrobials and improve practices at health facilities and within communities.

Keywords: antimicrobial resistance; antimicrobial stewardship; One Health approach

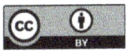

1. Project Overview

The partnership between Nottingham Trent University (NTU), Makerere University, Buckinghamshire Healthcare NHS Trust (BHT), and Entebbe Regional Referral Hospital (ERRH) has been promoting antimicrobial stewardship (AMS) in Wakiso District since 2019 using a One Health approach [1]. Other key stakeholders involved in this project include Wakiso district local government, the Ministry of Health, health practitioners, local leaders, and other policy makers. Various professionals including pharmacists, microbiologists, environmental health and public health scientists, and animal health experts have supported project activities.

Our most recent 7-month phase of the project, which ran from October 2021 to May 2022, was part of the Commonwealth Partnerships for Antimicrobial Stewardship (CwPAMS) grants. The project aimed to scale-up AMS interventions in Wakiso district, with a focus on capacity building, stakeholder engagement, and knowledge exchange using a One Health approach. Several activities were conducted, mainly at ERRH, including training eight pharmacy staff on conducting a Global Point Prevalence Survey (GPPS) [2]; collecting and analysing GPPS data; carrying out an AMS workshop among 24 members of the Medicines and Therapeutics Committee (MTC); holding a workshop among 25 laboratory staff and clinicians on AMS/antimicrobial resistance (AMR); developing a 2–3 year AMS action plan; providing mentorship support on AMS to five lower level health facilities; training 52 health practitioners (HPs) (community pharmacy staff, other human health, and animal health practitioners) and 151 community health workers (CHWs) on AMS, AMR, infection prevention and control (IPC), gender equality and social inclusion (GESI); and increasing membership/continuing to engage members of the earlier established Communities of Practice (COPs) on AMS for health professionals and students, which have grown to over 540 and 250 members, respectively.

Both the Uganda and UK teams were involved in co-designing and implementing the project interventions. The UK team facilitated AMS trainings and workshops virtually through blended learning. In addition, the UK team supported ERRH remotely in drafting the hospital's AMS Action Plan through online platforms such as Zoom for meetings and email for the review of documents. The Uganda team was involved in the day-to-day implementation of project activities.

2. Outcomes and Impact

We shared the project findings at the national One Health Technical Working Group (OHTWG) quarterly virtual meeting in March 2022 in Uganda. We also contributed to the education and awareness survey in the World Health Organization African region to inform regional education and awareness implementation from 2017 to 2021. During the GPPS at ERRH, four pharmacy interns, in addition to four hospital staff, were trained on data collection and analysis. The GPPS enabled ERRH to identify areas of improvement in AMS practice, and the upskilling of existing staff will contribute to the sustainability of interventions. In addition, the hospital staff attended an online GPPS training by the University of Antwerp, which made the in-person training more engaging and easy to understand for the participants.

By the end of the mentorship visits, all five lower level health facilities had formed AMS committees, selected AMS champions, and carried out health education on AMR/AMS among patients. Below is a quote from the project evaluation following the AMS mentorship sessions of a lower level health facility:

> The interventions suggested during the mentorship visits have been feasible among which was the creation of an AMS committee. We have also been guided about how we can reduce antimicrobial resistance. Previously, we did not know how to talk to patients but now with the different education materials we have, it is easier. We now have posters that increase awareness, and platforms from which we get information about AMS. We are very thankful for this mentorship by Entebbe Regional Referral Hospital.
>
> —Health officer in charge of a lower level health facility, Wakiso District.

Our training assessments showed that HPs and CHWs had gained more knowledge on AMR/AMS/IPC after the trainings. Of the 52 HPs who participated in the post-training assessment (File S1), 100% (52) correctly identified that antibiotics are effective against bacteria, compared to 78.8% (41/52) who had done so during the pre-training assessment. Meanwhile, out of the 151 CHWs who participated in the post-training assessment (File S2), 98.7% (149/151) reported that microorganisms can fail to respond to antimicrobials, compared to 49.7% (75/151) in the pre-training assessment. Overall, approximately 90% of ERRH staff, 95% of lower level health facility staff, and 98% of CHWs at our project sites have been trained on AMR/AMS/IPC. Furthermore, about 1,000 community members were reached and educated about AMS by the trained health practitioners, as established during the project evaluation. The human and animal health workers trained, as well as communities reached during the project, were empowered to act as change agents in their respective settings regarding the proper access and use of antimicrobials. Our project activities target all five objectives of Uganda's AMR National Action Plan related to: (1) public awareness, training, and education; (2) IPC; (3) the optimal access and use of antimicrobials; (4) surveillance; and (5) research and innovation, by providing local, measurable, and sustainable actions [3].

The BHT project pharmacy staff, who have had previous experience working on CwPAMS projects as a part of this health partnership, have taken on a mentorship role to support new pharmacists on the team. One pharmacist undertook the Chief Pharmaceutical Officer's Global Health Fellowship alongside their involvement in this project. The pharmacists have additionally been able to develop their leadership skills and knowledge of global health due to their engagement in ongoing activities [4]. The lessons learned through project activities have allowed the pharmacists to consider different methods and communication techniques for engaging with the public and working across sectors, which was helpful during the COVID-19 pandemic in the UK. Furthermore, the review of AMS materials for the training enabled the UK team to optimise resources for future activities both in Uganda and the UK.

3. Future Development

We hope to further scale-up project activities to reach other parts of Wakiso district and Uganda, enabling more health workers to be educated and take actions to support AMS. We also hope to educate more animal health practitioners on AMS, in order to raise awareness and strengthen the One Health approach of tackling AMR. As a means of ensuring the adoption of the AMS activities, we plan to engage behavioural specialists to consider how interventions implemented can be sustained at the facilities and within the community [5]. Our research and that of others has shown that many community members access antimicrobials without receiving a consultation from a health professional [6–8]. To combat this, we plan to expand the community engagement aspects of the project and training/increasing awareness among other community pharmacists and drug shop staff. In addition, we shall have further project dissemination to other local, national, and international audiences to have a wider impact. We shall also continue to seek more funding to carry out further AMS activities in Wakiso district and beyond.

Supplementary Materials: The following supporting information can be downloaded at: https://www.mdpi.com/article/10.3390/msf2022015007/s1, Figure S1: Poster presentation for scaling-up interventions for strengthening antimicrobial stewardship using a One Health approach in Wakiso district, Uganda; File S1: PDF on health practitioners' pre- and post-assessment report after training on AMR/AMS/IPC; File S2: PDF on community health workers' pre- and post-assessment report after training on AMS/ AMR/IPC.

Author Contributions: Conceptualization and methodology, D.M., C.B., J.W. and L.G.; project implementation: G.B.L., S.N., D.M., B.Y.N., C.B., F.N., F.E.K., J.G., K.R.-H., L.M., M.O.B. and L.G.; data collection and formal analysis, G.B.L., F.N., J.G., S.N. and D.M.; writing—original draft preparation, S.N., G.B.L. and D.M.; writing—review and editing, D.M., S.N., G.B.L., F.N., J.W., L.G., L.M., B.Y.N., C.B. and M.O.B.; funding acquisition, D.M., L.G. and C.B.; project administration, M.O.B., C.B., K.R.-H., B.Y.N., L.M., F.E.K., J.W., G.B.L. and S.N. All authors have read and agreed to the published version of the manuscript.

Funding: This research was funded under the Commonwealth Partnerships for Antimicrobial Stewardship (CwPAMS), an initiative of the Commonwealth Pharmacists Association (CPA) and Tropical Health and Education Trust (THET), under the Fleming Fund of the UK Department of Health and Social Care (DHSC), grant number CwE.B03; the APC was funded by the English Surveillance Programme for Antimicrobial Utilisation and Resistance (ESPAUR).

Institutional Review Board Statement: The study was conducted in accordance with the Declaration of Helsinki and approved by the Institutional Review Board of Makerere University College of Health Sciences, School of Health Sciences Research and Ethics Committee (MakSHS-REC) 2019-051, renewed on 2 December 2021 and registered at the Uganda National Council of Science and Technology (HS 2711) on 6 February 2020.

Informed Consent Statement: Written informed consent was obtained from all subjects involved in the study.

Data Availability Statement: Data are contained within the article or supplementary material. The data presented in this study are available in [File S1: PDF on health practitioners' pre- and post-assessment report after training on AMR/AMS/IPC; File S2: PDF on community health workers' pre- and post-assessment report after training on AMS/ AMR/IPC].

Acknowledgments: We acknowledge ERRH hospital administration and pharmacy department, especially Ismail Kizito Musoke and Jamawa Namusiri, for taking lead on the mentorship visits. Our field mobilizers Henry Bugembe and Henry Kajubi are much appreciated for their support during the training of community health workers. Wakiso district local government, especially the office of the District Health Officer and the Ministry of Health, is recognized for its continued support in the Makerere University research projects.

Conflicts of Interest: The authors declare no conflict of interest. The funders had no role in the design of the study; in the collection, analyses, or interpretation of data; in the writing of the manuscript; or in the decision to publish the results.

References

1. Musoke, D.; Kitutu, F.E.; Mugisha, L.; Amir, S.; Brandish, C.; Ikhile, D.; Kajumbula, H.; Kizito, I.M.; Lubega, G.B.; Niyongabo, F.; et al. A one health approach to strengthening antimicrobial stewardship in Wakiso District, Uganda. *Antibiotics* **2020**, *9*, 764. [CrossRef] [PubMed]
2. Sharing Global Knowledge. Supporting Local Actions. Available online: https://www.global-pps.com/ (accessed on 9 December 2022).
3. Uganda: Antimicrobial Resistance National Action Plan 2018–2023. Available online: https://www.who.int/publications/m/item/uganda-antimicrobial-resistance-national-action-plan-2018-2023 (accessed on 9 December 2022).
4. Brandish, C.; Garraghan, F.; Ng, B.Y.; Russell-Hobbs, K.; Olaoye, O.; Ashiru-Oredope, D. Assessing the impact of a Global Health Fellowship on pharmacists' leadership skills and consideration of benefits to the National Health Service (NHS) in the United Kingdom. *Healthcare* **2021**, *9*, 890. [CrossRef] [PubMed]
5. Byrne-Davis, L.M.T.; Bull, E.R.; Burton, A.; Dharni, N.; Gillison, F.; Maltinsky, W.; Mason, C.; Sharma, C.; Armitage, C.J.; Johnston, M.; et al. How behavioural science can contribute to health partnerships: The case of The Change Exchange. *Glob. Health* **2017**, *13*, 30. [CrossRef] [PubMed]
6. Musoke, D.; Namata, C.; Lubega, G.B.; Kitutu, F.E.; Mugisha, L.; Amir, S.; Brandish, C.; Gonza, J.; Ikhile, D.; Niyongabo, F.; et al. Access, use and disposal of antimicrobials among humans and animals in Wakiso district, Uganda: A qualitative study. *J. Pharm. Policy Pract.* **2021**, *14*, 69. [CrossRef] [PubMed]
7. Sakeena, M.H.F.; Bennett, A.A.; McLachlan, A.J. Non-prescription sales of antimicrobial agents at community pharmacies in developing countries: A systematic review. *Int. J. Antimicrob. Agents* **2018**, *52*, 771–782. [CrossRef] [PubMed]
8. Mukonzo, J.K.; Namuwenge, P.M.; Okure, G.; Mwesige, B.; Namusisi, O.K.; Mukanga, D. Over-the-counter suboptimal dispensing of antibiotics in Uganda. *J. Multidiscip. Healthc.* **2013**, *6*, 303–310. [CrossRef] [PubMed]

Disclaimer/Publisher's Note: The statements, opinions and data contained in all publications are solely those of the individual author(s) and contributor(s) and not of MDPI and/or the editor(s). MDPI and/or the editor(s) disclaim responsibility for any injury to people or property resulting from any ideas, methods, instructions or products referred to in the content.

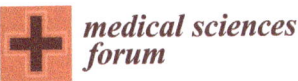

Proceeding Paper

Managing Penicillin Allergy in Primary Care: An Important but Neglected Aspect of Antibiotic Stewardship [†]

Marta Wanat [1,*], Sibyl Anthierens [2], Marta Santillo [1], Catherine Porter [3], Joanne Fielding [3], Mina Davoudianfar [1], Emily Bongard [1], Ly-Mee Yu [1], Christopher Butler [1], Louise Savic [4], Sinisa Savic [5], Johanna Cook [1], Kelsey Armitage [1], Philip Howard [6,7], Sue Pavitt [8], Jonathan A. T. Sandoe [3,‡] and Sarah Tonkin-Crine [1,9,‡]

1. Nuffield Department of Primary Care Health Sciences, University of Oxford, Oxford OX2 6GG, UK
2. Department of Family Medicine and Population Health, Faculty of Medicine and Health Sciences, University of Antwerp, 2610 Antwerp, Belgium
3. Healthcare Associated Infection Research Group, Leeds Institute of Medical Research, University of Leeds, Leeds LS2 9JT, UK
4. Department of Anaesthesia, Leeds Teaching Hospitals NHS Trust, Leeds LS1 3EX, UK
5. Department of Immunology and Allergy, Leeds Teaching Hospitals NHS Trust, Leeds LS1 3EX, UK
6. School of Healthcare, Faculty of Medicine and Health, University of Leeds, Leeds LS2 9JT, UK
7. Department of Medicines Management and Pharmacy, Leeds Teaching Hospitals NHS Trust, Leeds LS2 7UE, UK
8. Dental Translational and Clinical Research Unit, Faculty of Medicine and Health, University of Leeds, Leeds LS2 9JT, UK
9. National Institute for Health Research (NIHR) Health Protection Research Unit (HPRU) in Healthcare Associated Infections and Antimicrobial Resistance, University of Oxford, Oxford OX2 6GG, UK
* Correspondence: marta.wanat@phc.ox.ac.uk
† Presented at the 6th Antibiotic Guardian Shared Learning and Awards, Antibiotic Guardian, 2 May 2023; Available online: https://antibioticguardian.com/antibiotic-guardian-2022-shared-learning-awards/.
‡ Joint senior authors.

Abstract: An estimated 2.7 million people in the UK are potentially prevented from accessing highly effective and inexpensive penicillins as a result of incorrect penicillin allergy records. Removing incorrect penicillin allergy records may lead to improved patient outcomes and contribute to the tackling of antibiotic resistance. We aim to develop and evaluate whether the 'Penicillin Allergy Assessment Pathway' (PAAP) is effective in improving patient outcomes. At the first stage of this work, we have focused on understanding patients' and primary care clinicians' views of attending and referring to penicillin allergy testing, and then prescribing and consuming penicillin following a negative test result.

Keywords: penicillin allergy; general practice; intervention development

1. Project Overview

Penicillins are generally highly effective, narrow-spectrum, inexpensive antibiotics, and are the first-line recommended treatment for many infections. Around 6–10% of people in the UK have an allergy to penicillins listed in their medical records, but importantly, fewer than 1 in 10 of them are truly allergic [1]. This means that a significant proportion of patients are potentially restricted access to these highly effective penicillins. Incorrect penicillin allergy records are associated with antimicrobial resistance (AMR), as well as health outcomes (mortality, treatment failure, and surgical site infection) and altered antibiotic prescribing and resource use (e.g., longer hospital stays), and this is being recognised at the policy level. However, the management of penicillin allergy in primary care is challenging, as the awareness of and access to penicillin allergy testing is limited. We are conducting a programme of work that tries to address this gap. The initial stages of this programme involved a rapid review [2] and a qualitative study [3,4] with 31 patients and 19 primary

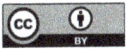

care physicians. This initial stage has allowed us to gain an in-depth understanding of the patient and primary care clinician views on managing penicillin allergy in primary care, and to identify the barriers and facilitators to penicillin allergy management and attending/referring for testing. These barriers were then mapped to behaviour change theories in order to describe the proposed mechanisms of change. Based on these findings, we have designed and developed behavioural intervention materials for both patients and clinicians to address their concerns and information needs. These intervention materials are now being used as a part of the 'ALABAMA' trial, targeting patients with a record of penicillin allergy deemed at low risk of true allergy. If the trial finds that this new approach to allergy assessment is effective and efficient, this would justify more patients being assessed and the allocation of appropriate resources. By incorporating behavioural science into safe and appropriate penicillin de-labelling, this work has the potential to significantly impact both direct patient care and the increasing burden of AMR.

2. Outcomes and Impact

The findings from our rapid review and qualitative study identified modifiable behavioural aspects, which were then systematically mapped onto the behaviour change theories. We have found that clinicians lacked experience of penicillin allergy testing services and thus wanted more information on what this testing involved and the safety of the tests, which, in turn, could help them to have conversations about testing with their patients [2–4]. The issue of safety was also described at length by patients, including their concerns about having a reaction, being adequately monitored during the test, the test invasiveness, and the safety of taking penicillins after a negative test [2–4]. We also found that both clinicians and patients did not perceive penicillin allergy to be a major problem in general practice due to the availability of alternative antibiotics [4]. Based on these findings, we have produced an intervention consisting of two booklets for patients and a handout for clinicians. Specifically, the 'Penicillin Allergy Testing: going for a test' leaflet for patients addresses the benefits of having access to penicillins and the safety of the test, while the 'Penicillin Allergy Testing: a negative test result' leaflet provides information about the accuracy of the testing and addresses patient concerns about consuming penicillins after a negative test. The clinician materials entitled 'Penicillin Allergy Testing: Information for general practice', contains information on penicillin allergy testing, the importance of de-labelling, and safety of the testing. These intervention materials are now being used as a part of the 'ALABAMA' trial, examining if a new pre-emptive 'penicillin allergy assessment pathway' that targets patients assessed as low risk of true allergy can be clinically effective in improving patient health outcomes and antibiotic use.

The importance of our findings has been acknowledged by the selection for the NIHR Evidence Alert as a study most likely to be of interest to the public and professionals, and to inform changes to policy and practice. The Alert highlighted the importance of checking penicillin allergy records and the further research needed in this area [5].

3. Future Development

If the "ALABAMA" trial finds that this new approach to allergy assessment is effective and efficient, this would justify more patients being assessed and the allocation of appropriate resources. This would have an impact on antibiotic prescribing and consumption, which are key components of antibiotic stewardship. Further interviews with patients and clinicians will examine the feasibility and acceptability of the PAAP and the materials, which will be crucial in ensuring the successful implementation of the pathway, if it is found effective.

Supplementary Materials: The following supporting information can be is downloaded at: https://www.mdpi.com/article/10.3390/msf2022015008/s1, Poster: Managing penicillin allergy in primary care: an important but neglected aspect of antibiotic stewardship.

Author Contributions: Conceptualization, J.A.T.S., C.B., S.P., S.S., L.S., E.B., P.H. and S.T.-C.; methodology, S.T.-C., S.A., M.W. and M.S.; formal analysis, S.T.-C., S.A., M.W. and M.S.; investigation, C.P., J.F., M.D., L.-M.Y., J.C. and K.A.; resources, J.A.T.S., C.B., S.P., S.S., L.S., E.B. and S.T.-C.; data curation, M.W.; writing—original draft preparation, M.W.; writing—review and editing, All; supervision, S.T.-C. and J.A.T.S.; project administration, J.F. and C.P.; funding acquisition, J.A.T.S., C.B., P.H., S.T.-C. and S.P. All authors have read and agreed to the published version of the manuscript.

Funding: This work was supported by the National Institute for Health Research (NIHR) under its Programme Grants for Applied Research Programme (Grant Number RP-PG-1214-20007) and by the National Institute for Health Research (NIHR) Health Protection Research Unit in Healthcare Associated Infections and Antimicrobial Resistance (NIHR200915) at the University of Oxford in partnership with the UK Health Security Agency (UKHSA) (ST-C and CCB) and by the National Institute for Health Research (NIHR) infrastructure at Leeds.

Institutional Review Board Statement: The study was conducted in accordance with the Declaration of Helsinki, and approved by the London Bridge Research Ethics Committee (Ref: 19/LO/0176).

Informed Consent Statement: Informed consent was obtained from all subjects involved in the study.

Data Availability Statement: Data are available upon reasonable request.

Conflicts of Interest: The funders had no role in the design of the study; in the collection, analyses, or interpretation of data; in the writing of the manuscript; or in the decision to publish the results.

References

1. Powell, N.; Kohl, D.; Ahmed, S.; Kent, B.; Sandoe, J.; Tonkin-Crine, S.; Owens, R.; Stephens, J.; Upton, M. Effectiveness of interventions that support penicillin allergy assessment and de-labeling of patients by non-allergy specialists: A systematic review protocol. *JBI Evid. Synth.* **2022**, *20*, 624–632. [CrossRef]
2. Wanat, M.; Anthierens, S.; Butler, C.C.; Wright, J.M.; Dracup, N.; Pavitt, S.H.; Sandoe, J.A.; Tonkin-Crine, S. Patient and prescriber views of penicillin allergy testing and subsequent antibiotic use: A rapid review. *Antibiotics* **2018**, *7*, 71. [CrossRef] [PubMed]
3. Wanat, M.; Anthierens, S.; Butler, C.C.; Savic, L.; Savic, S.; Pavitt, S.H.; Sandoe, J.A.; Tonkin-Crine, S. Patient and primary care physician perceptions of penicillin allergy testing and subsequent use of penicillin-containing antibiotics: A qualitative study. *J. Allergy Clin. Immunol. Pract.* **2019**, *7*, 1888–1893. [CrossRef]
4. Wanat, M.; Anthierens, S.; Butler, C.C.; Savic, L.; Savic, S.; Pavitt, S.H.; Sandoe, J.A.; Tonkin-Crine, S. Management of penicillin allergy in primary care: A qualitative study with patients and primary care physicians. *BMC Fam. Pract.* **2021**, *22*, 112. [CrossRef] [PubMed]
5. Are you Sure You Are Allergic to Penicillin? Professionals and Patients Are Urged to Double-Check. Available online: https://evidence.nihr.ac.uk/alert/are-you-sure-you-are-allergic-to-penicillin/ (accessed on 15 December 2022).

Disclaimer/Publisher's Note: The statements, opinions and data contained in all publications are solely those of the individual author(s) and contributor(s) and not of MDPI and/or the editor(s). MDPI and/or the editor(s) disclaim responsibility for any injury to people or property resulting from any ideas, methods, instructions or products referred to in the content.

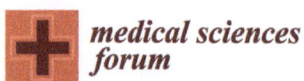 

Proceeding Paper

Informing Antibiotic Guardianship to Combat Antimicrobial Resistance: The Liverpool Citizens' Jury on AMR [†]

William Hope [1,*], James Amos [2], Sarah Atwood [3], Kyle Bozentko [3], Amanda Lamb [1], Gary Leeming [1], Matthew Smith [4], Rachel Thompson [1] and Andrew Townsend [4]

[1] Faculty of Health and Life Sciences, University of Liverpool, Liverpool L3 5RT, UK
[2] Pfizer Limited, Kent CT13 9NJ, UK
[3] Center for New Democratic Processes, MN 55101, USA
[4] Pfizer Inc., New York, NY 10017, USA
* Correspondence: hopew@liverpool.ac.uk
† Presented at the 6th Antibiotic Guardian Shared Learning and Awards, Antibiotic Guardian, 2 May 2023; Available online: https://antibioticguardian.com/antibiotic-guardian-2022-shared-learning-awards/.

Abstract: The Liverpool Citizens' Jury was a public consultation on the use of health data to tackle the significant problem of Antimicrobial Resistance (AMR) and is the first step in creating a local AMR network with national and international relevance. The 18 jurors were tasked with learning about AMR as it relates to research and considered how organisations might collect, share and utilise pseudo-anonymised patient data. The overarching aim is to produce a new model supporting societal change focused on Antibiotic Guardianship and to combat the public health challenge of AMR. The model will be implemented in the UK and provided to an international network enabling global knowledge transfer.

Keywords: citizen jury; public engagement; deliberative democracy; AMR; antimicrobial resistance; data; health data; pharmaceuticals; Liverpool; Liverpool City Region

1. Project Overview

This study was conducted as a collaboration between the University of Liverpool, the Center for New Democratic Processes and Pfizer Inc. The University of Liverpool and Pfizer Inc. were the study sponsors.

This Citizens' Jury project was a public engagement event that formed the basis of the consultation stage of phase 1 of a multi-year programme of work to develop a better information and data sharing model for Antibiotic Guardianship. The first consultation was delivered using the deliberative method of a Citizen Jury. The jury (wherein people are recruited to broadly reflect the demographics of a particular catchment area) were asked to hear and weigh the evidence, discuss together, and use their values to assess trade-offs and make judgements regarding their remit.

The evidence came from a range of expert witnesses who had been briefed to create presentations that provide the jury with a fair balance of relevant information. Over two weeks, jurors encountered and engaged with a series of frameworks to assess the challenge(s) at hand, learnt from presenters, and worked collaboratively to assess the benefits and trade-offs of proposed solutions. They made informed recommendations regarding the legal, ethical, and regulatory aspects of the proposal.

The jurors considered patients in hospital with confirmed urinary tract infections (UTI) who were prescribed different antimicrobial regimens by their healthcare practitioners. They were then asked questions based on the scenario to provide an understanding of the public perceptions of information and data access that required for optimal use of newly approved drugs and treatments.

Jurors were generally supportive of the sharing of health data for AMR research, although support varied depending upon the activity and the parties involved. When considering hospital staff use of data, jurors indicated 95% support for data use to identify trends in AMR manifesting in serious illness. When asked the same question about researcher and pharmaceutical companies using health data to investigate trends in AMR, jurors indicated 84% and 89% support, respectively. However, only 56% of jurors supported government researchers using data to analyse trends in AMR [1].

The jurors identified five areas for future consideration as the project progresses. These were: access to data, acquiring consent for data use, quality of data use, security of data and use of data [2] (pp. 25–26).

Jurors generally indicated that they found the jury a positive experience, with 100% answering that they found the jury process 'very interesting' when polled in the final jury session [2] (p. 30). Jurors were quoted as saying,

> "Hopefully the work we have done will go towards a very positive and important project of finding an answer to AMR. This project is the brainchild of people in our Merseyside region and it's good to see that we could be having such an input into the future health of the country and the world as a whole [1] (p. 3)".

> "Having listened to a number of presentations from esteemed professionals, we have collaborated as a 'Jury' to express our views on proposals to use and share personal data for the purposes of addressing this important area of public health. Put simply, it is to try and find solutions to the fact that antibiotics are becoming less effective and we need to research, fund and find new treatments and drugs for the benefit of us all. Our findings will help shape policy to address these issues [1] (p. 33)".

The whole process was facilitated by a third party, the Center for New Democratic Processes, and was overseen by an independent panel whose purpose was to ensure fairness in the information provided to the jury. They worked with the jury to provide a safe space to express opinions and concerns. The jury produced a final report complete with recommendations for the next stages of the project and this was presented back to the project team, which was accepted in its entirety.

2. Outcomes and Impact

2.1. Citizen AMR Champions and AMR Awareness

Delivery of the event stimulated conversations on social media (Twitter, LinkedIn) about AMR, raising the profile locally and nationally. Follower counts on social channels increased considerably, and impression counts were in the top quartile of similar posts. Additionally, the event raised the importance of meaningful public involvement in research across the research and development community.

The 18 members of the jury received significant education on a broad range of topics related to AMR, drug development and legal and ethical considerations of data usage. Consequentially, they are extremely enthusiastic to champion Guardianship more broadly, with one juror explaining how this experience "has changed my life for the better".

2.2. Knowledge Exchange

All materials, slides and presentations for the event were produced by leading experts in their field, were assessed by an oversight panel to address any perceived bias and written for a lay audience. Distillation of the results was published in a series of reports and all raw data are available. A dedicated webpage is hosted by the University of Liverpool to hold all assets, which are freely accessible.

2.3. Understanding Public Perception

The key outputs were gaining insight into what the public thought about:

- The visibility of AMR and AMR research;
- What information the public would like to see about AMR;
- Which sources of information are trusted by the public;
- Public and private sector organisations accessing data;
- Public and private partnerships working together;
- What legal, ethical and regulatory considerations they most value.

These insights will be incorporated into the ongoing work and will enable the co-development of a framework that will support a community to become Antibiotic Guardians.

3. Future Development

The Citizens' Jury project forms the basis of the consultation stage of phase 1 of a multi-year programme of work to develop a better information and data sharing model for Antibiotic Guardianship. The learnings from public perceptions are currently being incorporated into the initial programme design. Changes have already been made in terms of the ways of working, the level and types of outreach work and an emphasis on explaining process as well as outcomes. The Jury told us that clear communication on data use was something that helped with the building of trust and displaying of trustworthiness. The public involvement section of the programme will be significantly expanded to enable repeated involvement of the public in further iterations of the design and implementation processes.

Nationally and internationally, we have been developing an expansive network to ensure that the knowledge gained from this exercise is reused and starts to form the foundations of a better way of involving the public at the heart of system design. However, some of the recommendations of the jury have already been implemented and guided similar projects in Liverpool that use connected health data.

Supplementary Materials: The following supporting information can be downloaded at: https://www.mdpi.com/article/10.3390/msf2022015009/s1, Conference Poster: A new model to inform Antibiotic Guardianship and combat Antimicrobial Resistance: The Liverpool Citizens' Jury.

Author Contributions: Conceptualization, J.A., S.A., K.B., W.H., A.L., G.L., M.S., R.T. and A.T.; methodology, S.A. and K.B.; formal analysis, S.A. and K.B.; investigation, S.A. and K.B.; resources, S.A. and K.B.; data curation, S.A. and K.B.; writing—original draft preparation, J.A., S.A., K.B., W.H., A.L., M.S., R.T. and A.T.; writing—review and editing, J.A., S.A., K.B., A.L., R.T. and A.T.; supervision, W.H. and A.L.; project administration, A.L. and R.T.; funding acquisition, W.H., A.L. and G.L. All authors have read and agreed to the published version of the manuscript.

Funding: This initiative was funded by Pfizer Inc. 'Smart Antimicrobial Systems (SAS) to provide actionable information to tackle Antimicrobial Resistance grant (CEIDR-Pfizer-SAS-2021), and by Liverpool City Region Combined Authority in the 'Civic Data Cooperative' grant (LCR-CDC-UOL-162335).

Institutional Review Board Statement: Ethical review and approval were waived for this study as it was deemed by the University of Liverpool as public engagement and not research.

Informed Consent Statement: Informed consent was obtained from all subjects involved in the public engagement event.

Data Availability Statement: The data presented in this study are available in https://www.liverpool.ac.uk/media/livacuk/iib/AMR_Full,Report_Final,V1.4.pdf.

Acknowledgments: Many thanks to the members of the public who acted as jurors during this project. Thanks should also go to the AMR Citizens' Jury Oversight Panel and the expert witnesses.

Conflicts of Interest: The authors declare no conflict of interest. Funders were not involved in the study design or management of the Citizens' Jury process.

References

1. Liverpool AMR Citizens' Jury Full Report. Available online: https://www.liverpool.ac.uk/media/livacuk/iib/AMR_Full, Report_Final,V1.4.pdf (accessed on 10 December 2022).
2. Liverpool AMR Citizens' Jury Executive Summary. Available online: https://www.liverpool.ac.uk/media/livacuk/iib/AMR_Executive_Summary_Final,v1.4.pdf (accessed on 10 December 2022).

Disclaimer/Publisher's Note: The statements, opinions and data contained in all publications are solely those of the individual author(s) and contributor(s) and not of MDPI and/or the editor(s). MDPI and/or the editor(s) disclaim responsibility for any injury to people or property resulting from any ideas, methods, instructions or products referred to in the content.

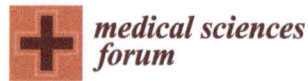 

Proceeding Paper

Developing a Board and Online Game to Educate People on Antimicrobial Resistance and Stewardship: The AMS Game [†]

Sarah Cavanagh [1], Frances Garraghan [1,*], Maxencia Nabiryo [1,*], Diane Ashiru-Oredope [1], Melvin Bell [2] and Victoria Rutter [1]

[1] Commonwealth Pharmacists Association, London E1W 1AW, UK
[2] Focus Games, Glasgow G40 1DA, UK
* Correspondence: frances.garraghan@commonwealthpharmacy.org (F.G.); maxencia.nabiryo@commonwealthpharmacy.org (M.N.)
[†] Presented at the 6th Antibiotic Guardian Shared Learning and Awards, Antibiotic Guardian, 2 May 2023; Available online: https://antibioticguardian.com/antibiotic-guardian-2022-shared-learning-awards/.

Abstract: To support efforts towards addressing the increasingly growing global burden of antimicrobial resistance (AMR), a diverse and multicountry team of stakeholders developed a board and online game on antimicrobial stewardship (AMS). The game aims to create awareness and develop knowledge of healthcare teams at all levels. Reports from initial players reflect that the game is an innovative, engaging and inclusive education resource on AMR and AMS. The game continues to be promoted for continued and wider usage across the globe.

Keywords: AMS game; Commonwealth Partnerships for Antimicrobial Stewardship; CwPAMS; antimicrobial resistance (AMR); antimicrobial stewardship (AMS); board game; game-based learning; gamification; gaming; online game

1. Project Overview

Innovative, effective training and skills building are vital to the success of antimicrobial stewardship (AMS) programmes, particularly when staff are new to the concept. The AMS game is a digital and physical board game intended to make AMS training engaging and inclusive, generating fun and enthusiasm, with educative purposes and outcomes.

2. Outcomes and Impact

The game was co-created with a diverse group of stakeholders from high-and low-income countries. The feedback from the initial players of the game highlighted that the game is enjoyable and provides an innovative and engaging opportunity to discuss AMR and AMS, whilst improving and strengthening their knowledge of key topics. There are sustainability and global impacts of the use of digital/online games and the "buy one, donate one" rollout model.

3. Future Development

The AMS Game is an established tool in the Commonwealth Pharmacists Association's AMR programme activities, enabling the promotion of the game in training across the Commonwealth and beyond. This will be promoted and expanded globally via the second phase of the Commonwealth Partnerships for Antimicrobial Stewardship (CwPAMS 2) programme. In addition, given the constraints on NHS training budgets, the game will be promoted as a cost-effective training resource throughout the UK. The game will be updated based on feedback and best practice. In 2023, outreach will be expanded into India with a Hindi translation of the game.

Citation: Cavanagh, S.; Garraghan, F.; Nabiryo, M.; Ashiru-Oredope, D.; Bell, M.; Rutter, V. Developing a Board and Online Game to Educate People on Antimicrobial Resistance and Stewardship: The AMS Game. *Med. Sci. Forum* **2022**, *15*, 12. https://doi.org/10.3390/msf2022015012

Academic Editor: Jordan Charlesworth

Published: 24 March 2023

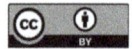

Copyright: © 2023 by the authors. Licensee MDPI, Basel, Switzerland. This article is an open access article distributed under the terms and conditions of the Creative Commons Attribution (CC BY) license (https://creativecommons.org/licenses/by/4.0/).

Supplementary Materials: The material is available at https://www.mdpi.com/article/10.3390/msf2022015012/s1, Conference Poster: Developing a Board and Online Game to Educate on Antimicrobial Resistance and Stewardship.

Author Contributions: Conceptualization, F.G., D.A.-O. and S.C.; data curation, F.G., M.N., S.C., D.A.-O. and M.B.; methodology, F.G., M.N. and D.A.-O.; project administration, M.N., S.C., M.B. and F.G.; supervision, F.G.; validation, F.G.; writing—original draft, F.G., S.C. and M.N.; writing—review and editing, D.A.-O., M.N., M.B., S.C., F.G. and V.R. All authors have read and agreed to the published version of the manuscript.

Funding: This project and partnership were part of the Commonwealth Partnerships for Antimicrobial Stewardship (CwPAMS) managed by the Tropical Health and Education Trust (THET) and Commonwealth Pharmacists Association (CPA). CwPAMS is a global health partnership programme funded by the Department of Health and Social Care (DHSC) using UK aid funding. The views expressed in this publication are those of the authors and not necessarily those of the DHSC or its Management Agent, Mott MacDonald, the UK National Health Service, the Tropical Health and Education Trust, or the Commonwealth Pharmacists Association.

Institutional Review Board Statement: Ethical approval was not required as per NHS Health Research Authority guidance and the NHS health research decision tool because this was a service evaluation of CPA's programme of activities to develop and implement the AMS game as part of the CwPAMS programme. All respondents participated strictly in their professional capacity, no identifiable data were collected, and their participation in the survey was in all cases on the basis of informed consent.

Informed Consent Statement: Informed consent was obtained from all participants involved in the study.

Data Availability Statement: Data are contained within the article or Supplementary Material.

Acknowledgments: Project team: Diane Ashiru-Oredope, Nikki D'Arcy, Will Townsend, Sarah Cavanagh, Richard Skone-James, Frances Garraghan, and Melvin Bell. Many thanks to all who were involved in the development process. For more information visit www.amsgame.com.

Conflicts of Interest: The authors declare no conflict of interest. The funders had no role in the design of the study; in the collection, analyses, or interpretation of data; in the writing of the manuscript; or in the decision to publish the results.

Disclaimer/Publisher's Note: The statements, opinions and data contained in all publications are solely those of the individual author(s) and contributor(s) and not of MDPI and/or the editor(s). MDPI and/or the editor(s) disclaim responsibility for any injury to people or property resulting from any ideas, methods, instructions or products referred to in the content.

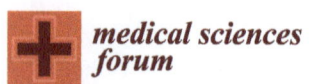

Proceeding Paper

Engaging the Global Dental Profession to Help Tackle Antibiotic Resistance [†]

Paula Anabalon-Cordova [1], Susie Sanderson [1], David Williams [2], Mahesh Verma [3], Céline Pulcini [4], Leanne Teoh [5] and Wendy Thompson [6,*]

1. Education and Public Health, FDI World Dental Federation, 1216 Geneva, Switzerland
2. Institute of Dentistry, Queen Mary University of London, London E1 2HA, UK
3. Maulana Azad Institute of Dental Sciences, Delhi University, New Delhi 110002, India
4. Research Unit 4360 APEMAC, Université de Lorraine, BP 20199, 54505 Nancy, France
5. Melbourne Dental School, University of Melbourne, Carlton, VIC 3053, Australia
6. Division of Dentistry, University of Manchester, Manchester M13 9PL, UK
* Correspondence: wendy.thompson15@nhs.net
† Presented at the 6th Antibiotic Guardian Shared Learning and Awards, Antibiotic Guardian, 2 May 2023; Available online: https://antibioticguardian.com/antibiotic-guardian-2022-shared-learning-awards/.

Abstract: In the pre-antibiotic era, deaths from dental infections were common. Dentists are responsible for prescribing around 10% of antibiotics across healthcare globally. During 2020, dental antibiotic prescribing increased dramatically due to COVID-19 pandemic restrictions on dental procedures, which are vital for preventing and managing dental infections. FDI World Dental Federation responded with a framework about the essential role of dental teams in tackling antibiotic resistance, setting out a program to engage the global dental profession. Three exemplars include an open online course (with >2300 learners enrolled from >100 countries), a pledge for national dental organizations, and an early career researcher network.

Keywords: dental care; oral health; antibiotic; antimicrobial; resistance; engagement; communication

Citation: Anabalon-Cordova, P.; Sanderson, S.; Williams, D.; Verma, M.; Pulcini, C.; Teoh, L.; Thompson, W. Engaging the Global Dental Profession to Help Tackle Antibiotic Resistance. *Med. Sci. Forum* **2022**, *15*, 13. https://doi.org/10.3390/msf2022015013

Academic Editor: Diane Ashiru-Oredope

Published: 24 March 2023

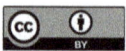

Copyright: © 2023 by the authors. Licensee MDPI, Basel, Switzerland. This article is an open access article distributed under the terms and conditions of the Creative Commons Attribution (CC BY) license (https://creativecommons.org/licenses/by/4.0/).

1. Project Overview

"Rotten teeth are rarely life-threatening, thanks to antibiotics" [1]. In the pre-antibiotic era, however, death from oral and dental infections were common [2]. Dentists are responsible for around 10% of antibiotic prescribing across human healthcare globally [3].

During 2020, dental antibiotic prescribing increased dramatically due to COVID-19 pandemic restrictions on dental procedures to prevent and manage dental infections [4]. In response, FDI World Dental Federation (Geneva, Switzerland) published a framework about the essential role of dental teams in tackling antibiotic resistance [3]. Aligned with the World Health Organization (WHO) (Geneva, Switzerland) Global Action Plan's objectives [5], its recommendations aim to raise awareness, prevent infections, and optimise the use of antibiotics in dentistry, including by building the capacity of the global research base for dental antibiotic prescribing, resistance, and stewardship. To accompany its launch, an online library of resources which can be tailored to the local context was published [6], along with an open online course [7].

FDI is the main representative body for more than one million dentists worldwide. Its membership comprises some 200 national member associations and specialist groups in over 130 countries. In addition to the exemplar projects described in the following sections, FDI continues to engage and communicate about dental antibiotics globally, including through professional webinars [8], courses [7], and conferences [9], as well as with the wider public through media releases [10] and online videos [11] via World Dental Congress [9], AMR Youth Summit, International Association for Dental Research [12], and FDI's Oral Health Campus [8].

Three exemplars are presented to demonstrate the impact so far of FDI's framework and how it has been embedded across the dental community globally: at the clinical (dental team and patient) level via national dental associations, and with academia. These include an open online course [7], a pledge for national dental organisations [13], and a network for early career researchers [14].

2. Outcomes and Impact

2.1. Engaging with Individuals

Accompanying the FDI white paper [3] is an open online course developed collaboratively with Future Learn and the British Society for Antimicrobial Chemotherapy (BSAC) [7]. Since its launch during World Antimicrobial Awareness Week (WAAW) 2020, more than 2300 learners have enrolled from more than 100 countries, including 61 Global South countries. Designed to provide something for everyone whilst recognising the breadth of experience and differences in local contexts, FDI is delighted with the course's popularity among dental students (from Afghanistan, Bolivia, Mongolia, and many more countries), aspiring dental students, and the wider public.

2.2. Commitment of National Organizations

FDI's white paper [3] encourages National Dental Associations (NDAs) and other organisations to commit to tackling antibiotic resistance, to advocate for dentistry within national action plans on antimicrobial resistance (AMR), and to support members of the profession to use antibiotics responsibly. To support delivery of this goal, FDI produced a pledge for them to tackle antibiotic resistance by implementing local activities, such as raising awareness, preventing dental infections and optimising antibiotic prescribing [13]. Launched during WAAW 2021, more than 60 NDAs and 50 other dental organisations/individuals have signed so far.

2.3. Capacity of Researchers

At the International Association for Dental Research (IADR) 2021, FDI launched its Global Antimicrobial Research in Dentistry (GARD) early career researcher network. Its aim is to build capacity for research on dental antimicrobial prescribing, resistance, and stewardship, and it already has over 100 members from around the world, including pharmacists, infectious disease specialists, and, of course, dentists. Details of its monthly online journal club are advertised via its LinkedIn forum. At these lively Zoom events, volunteers present their recent research (with 20 presentations so far) and ideas for future collaborations are generated. The results of one such study reviewing guidelines in Latin America were presented at IADR 2022 [12]. Another study involved co-developing international consensus on a core outcome set for dental antibiotic stewardship with patients, clinicians, and academics participating in the study [15].

3. Future Development

3.1. Engaging the Public

Responding to feedback from the online course, a set of resources highlighting the benefits of managing dental pain and infection without antibiotics will aim to reduce professional intention to prescribe, and public desire for, antibiotics by tackling the erroneous yet widespread perception that antibiotics are necessary and appropriate for treating acute dental problems [16]. FDI intends to produce awareness-raising posters, leaflets and videos which can be used globally. Template resources for member National Dental Associations and other partners will also be provided, which can be adapted to address local problems, such as over-the-counter access to antibiotics [17].

3.2. National and International Action

FDI will continue to use its influence to encourage the inclusion of dentistry within national action plans on AMR and vice versa (AMR within oral health plans). FDI is particularly pleased that the WHO recently incorporated AMR into its global oral health action plan, and more recently its Global Oral Health Status Report 2022 [18].

World Dental Congress Sydney 2023 will be the first in-person event since the white paper's publication. A celebratory event for signatories of FDI's pledge is planned to publicly share their successes and encourage a wider range of signatories, including from South America, Africa, businesses, and charities involved with dentistry.

3.3. Collaborative Research and Mentoring

International collaborative research through the GARD network will be our future focus for active engagement with academic stakeholders. Network members will be involved with disseminating the results of our studies, including the review of Latin American guidelines [12] and the international consensus on a core outcome set for dental antibiotic stewardship [15] once they are published. Collaboration has also commenced on an international survey to identify patterns of practice and attitudes towards antibiotic prophylaxis for surgical site infections following dental procedures. This will be the first project to benefit from the network's mentoring programme.

In addition, an IADR symposium proposal on noma was conceived during a GARD journal club. This life-threatening tropical disease starts as an oral infection in severely malnourished children, and without effective antibiotic treatment is fatal in 90% of cases. The noma symposium has been accepted for the IADR General Session 2023, Bogota, Colombia.

Supplementary Materials: A poster to showcase how FDI's antibiotic stewardship program engaged the global dental profession is presented as Supplementary Material. The poster is available at https://www.mdpi.com/article/10.3390/msf2022015013/s1, Poster: Engaging the global dental profession to help tackle antibiotic resistance.

Author Contributions: Conceptualization, P.A.-C., S.S., D.W. and W.T.; writing—original draft preparation, W.T.; supervision, W.T., D.W., S.S., M.V. and C.P.; project administration, P.A.-C. and L.T.; funding acquisition, P.A.-C. and S.S. All authors have read and agreed to the published version of the manuscript.

Funding: This research was funded, in part, by GSK Healthcare.

Informed Consent Statement: Not applicable.

Data Availability Statement: Not applicable.

Acknowledgments: To the national dental associations who have actively delivered FDI's program.

Conflicts of Interest: The authors declare no conflict of interest. The funder had no role in the design of the program, in the writing of the manuscript, or in the decision to publish these proceedings.

References

1. The Guardian View on the Dentist Shortage: A Gap That Needs Filling. Available online: https://www.theguardian.com/commentisfree/2022/may/02/the-guardian-view-on-the-dentist-shortage-a-gap-that-needs-filling (accessed on 19 December 2022).
2. Appleby, J.; Stahl-Timmins, W. Consumption, flux, and dropsy: Counting deaths in 17th century London. *Br. Med. J.* **2018**, *363*, k5014. [CrossRef]
3. Thompson, W.; Williams, D.; Pulcini, C.; Sanderson, S.; Calfon, P.; Verma, M. *The Essential Role of the Dental Team in Reducing Antibiotic Resistance*; FDI World Dental Federation: Geneva, Switzerland, 2020.
4. Shah, S.; Wordley, V.; Thompson, W. How did COVID-19 impact on dental antibiotic prescribing across England? *Br. Dent. J.* **2020**, *229*, 601–604. [CrossRef] [PubMed]
5. World Health Organization. *Global Action Plan on Antimicrobial Resistance*; World Health Organization: Geneva, Switzerland, 2015.
6. Antibiotic Stewardship for Dental Teams: A Library of Resources. Available online: https://fdiforum.bsac.org.uk/ (accessed on 19 December 2022).
7. Tackling Antibiotic Resistance: What Should Dental Teams Do? Available online: www.futurelearn.com/courses/tackling-antibiotic-resistance-dentists (accessed on 19 December 2022).
8. Tackling Antibiotic Resistance: What Can the Dental Profession Do? Available online: www.fdioralhealthcampus.org/webinar/tackling-antibiotic-resistance-what-can-the-dental-profession-do/ (accessed on 19 December 2022).

9. "Infections Pay No Respect to Borders": Spotlight on ADA FDI World Dental Congress Speaker Dr Wendy Thompson. Available online: www.fdiworlddental.org/infections-pay-no-respect-borders-spotlight-ada-fdi-world-dental-congress-speaker-dr-wendy-thompson (accessed on 19 December 2022).
10. Prescribing of Dental Antibiotics up 22% in England during First Year of COVID-19. Available online: https://www.fdiworlddental.org/prescribing-dental-antibiotics-22-england-during-first-year-covid-19 (accessed on 19 December 2022).
11. FDI Team "Goes Blue for AMR" Because Antibiotic Resistance Is Everyone's Problem. Available online: www.fdiworlddental.org/fdi-team-goes-blue-amr-because-antibiotic-resistance-everyones-problem (accessed on 19 December 2022).
12. Thompson, W.; Teoh, L.; Anabalon-Cordova, P. Antimicrobial resistance and COVID-19: Two pandemics. In Proceedings of the International Association for Dental Research General Session 2022, Online, 20–25 June 2022.
13. Antibiotic Resistance Needs Tackling Immediately Across Dentistry: Sign the Pledge. Available online: www.fdiworlddental.org/antibiotic-resistance-needs-tackling-immediately-across-dentistry (accessed on 19 December 2022).
14. GARD Early Career Researcher Network. Available online: https://www.fdiworlddental.org/global-antimicrobial-resistance-dental-gard-early-career-researcher-network (accessed on 19 December 2022).
15. Thompson, W.; Teoh, L.; Pulcini, C.; Williams, D.; Pitkeathley, C.; Carter, V.; Sanderson, S.; Torres, G.; Walsh, T. Dental antibiotic stewardship: Study protocol for developing international consensus on a core outcome set. *Trials* **2022**, *23*, 116. [CrossRef] [PubMed]
16. Emmott, R.; Barber, S.K.; Thompson, W. Antibiotics and toothache: A social media review. *Int. J. Pharm Pract.* **2021**, *29*, 210–217. [CrossRef]
17. Sneddon, J.; Thompson, W.; Kpobi, L.N.; Ade, D.A.; Sefah, I.A.; Afriyie, D.; Goldthorpe, J.; Turner, R.; Nawaz, S.; Wilson, S.; et al. Exploring the use of antibiotics for dental patients in a middle-income country: Interviews with clinicians in two Ghanaian hospitals. *Antibiotics* **2022**, *11*, 1081. [CrossRef] [PubMed]
18. World Health Organization. *Global Oral Health Status Report: Towards Universal Health Coverage for Oral Health by 2030*; World Health Organization: Geneva, Switzerland, 2022.

Disclaimer/Publisher's Note: The statements, opinions and data contained in all publications are solely those of the individual author(s) and contributor(s) and not of MDPI and/or the editor(s). MDPI and/or the editor(s) disclaim responsibility for any injury to people or property resulting from any ideas, methods, instructions or products referred to in the content.

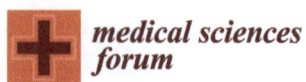 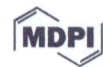

Proceeding Paper

Supporting Correct Antimicrobial Choices in Sepsis †

Balwinder Bolla [1],* and Alex Rond-Alliston [2]

[1] Department of Pharmacy, United Lincolnshire Hospitals, Lincoln LN25QY, UK
[2] East Cheshire NHS Trust, Macclesfield SK10 3BL, UK
* Correspondence: balwinder.bolla@ulh.nhs.uk; Tel.: +44-01522-573735
† Presented at the 6th Antibiotic Guardian Shared Learning and Awards, Antibiotic Guardian, 2 May 2023; Available online: https://antibioticguardian.com/antibiotic-guardian-2022-shared-learning-awards/.

Abstract: Antimicrobial audits on A&E and acute admissions wards have highlighted deficiencies in prescribing practices, particularly the inappropriate use of broad-spectrum agents. A clinical decision-making tool was created to expedite and facilitate the process of selecting correct antimicrobial treatments based on the site and severity of an infection, and also included the consideration of penicillin allergy. Simple, efficient, and effective, this tool has already been shared with many NHS Trusts nationally. Further audits, after this tool was introduced, show improvements in some aspects of antimicrobial prescribing, despite limited opportunities to deliver an awareness campaign of this resource. Such action will be needed to drive further improvements in antimicrobial prescribing choices in sepsis.

Keywords: antibiotic; antimicrobial; stewardship; prescriptions; clinical decision tool; broad-spectrum antibiotics; sepsis; allergy

1. Project Overview

Several reasons to improve the awareness of correct antimicrobial choices in sepsis have been highlighted in our Trust. These range from mortality risk and significant side effects to more widespread inappropriate escalations of antibiotics or inadequate cover provided by choices.

Antibiotic stewardship is vital to try to limit the growth of antimicrobial resistance, which has been described as one of the WHO's top ten global public health threats [1] and is responsible for more than 50,000 bloodstream infections each year in the UK, with considerable associated mortality [2].

Antimicrobial audits undertaken in our A&E department and on acute surgical wards have revealed the inappropriate use of broad-spectrum antibiotics, particularly piperacillin–tazobactam and meropenem. Two key issues were highlighted by root cause analyses:

1. Incorrect labeling of localized infectious disease as sepsis.
2. Perception of poor differentiation of treatment choices in current guidelines, even where there is a clear suspected cause.

The existing antimicrobial guidance and posters were felt to be unclear and difficult to read due to the volume of information.

The purpose of creating a new clinical decision-making tool was to improve both the access and clarity of Trusts' antimicrobial recommendations in sepsis, sources known and unknown, that can be referred to swiftly at the point of prescribing. These recommendations need to be clear, concise, and easily used in daily practice.

This tool (Figure S2) simplifies the choice of antimicrobials required by way of a few simple questions, with clarification and further information if required by a user. It easily can, and has, been updated to reflect changes to guidelines, ensuring that it remains relevant to local antimicrobial trends.

2. Outcomes and Impact

The tool has seen widespread use since its creation and adoption (Figure S3). Its use has increased with time, with the greatest use being seen during the junior doctor turnover month of August, helping new prescribers to familiarize themselves with local guidelines. It has received positive feedback from staff, particularly regarding its ease of use, accessibility, and educational value, enabling rapid decisions and bolstering confidence in these decisions. Due to widespread interest, this tool has been shared with over a dozen hospitals and NHS Trusts in the UK (Figure S4).

A comparison of antimicrobial audit data has been undertaken for A&E in terms of the quality of prescribing prior to and after the introduction of this clinical decision tool (Table S1). Improvements in antimicrobial prescription practices in regard to the clarity of a site and the severity of an infection are notable. This may be attributed, in part, to the additional information provided in the tool. There was no indication of an improvement in the correct choice of antimicrobials at this point; however, the audits did not focus on sepsis presentation alone, as they were undertaken for multiple reasons. It is also important to state that the awareness campaign for this tool has not been optimized as of yet. Educational sessions, written communications, and walk-arounds have helped raise awareness, but in areas with high levels of agency and locum staffing more is needed to embed the message.

3. Future Development

Plans for this tool include increasing awareness with larger and timely educational campaigns, collating further feedback for the improvement of the next version, and views on how to maximize accessibility as well as convenience. Other work will include developing a bitesize educational video to accompany this tool and updating guidelines and posters with a direct QR code (Figure S2). Further surveillance of utilization and comparing audits will also be helpful in establishing how these efforts are progressing improvements in practice.

Supplementary Materials: The following supporting information can be downloaded at: https://www.mdpi.com/article/10.3390/msf2022015005/s1, Figure S1: Poster overview of the project; Figure S2: Screenshot of the tool itself, as viewed by a user. Note also the QR code in the bottom-right-hand corner to view the current version directly; Figure S3: Graph depicting the use of the tool in 2022 so far. Updated since poster submission for accuracy; Figure S4: List of hospitals and NHS Trusts that the tool has been shared with; Table S1: Overview of pre- and post-intervention audit data.

Author Contributions: Conceptualization, B.B.; methodology, B.B.; software, A.R.-A.; validation, B.B. and A.R.-A.; writing—original draft preparation, A.R.-A.; writing—review and editing, B.B. and A.R.-A.; visualization, A.R.-A. and B.B.; supervision, B.B. All authors have read and agreed to the published version of the manuscript.

Funding: This research received no external funding.

Institutional Review Board Statement: Not applicable.

Informed Consent Statement: Not applicable.

Data Availability Statement: The data presented in this study are available in Figures S1–S4 and Table S1.

Acknowledgments: The authors would like to thank Induction Guidance for developing the platform that enabled the development of this clinical decision tool.

Conflicts of Interest: The authors declare no conflict of interest.

References

1. Antimicrobial Resistance. Available online: https://www.who.int/news-room/fact-sheets/detail/antimicrobial-resistance (accessed on 16 December 2022).
2. Mahase, E. Changes in behaviour last year led to fall in antibiotic resistant infections. *BMJ* **2021**, *375*, n2853. [CrossRef] [PubMed]

Disclaimer/Publisher's Note: The statements, opinions and data contained in all publications are solely those of the individual author(s) and contributor(s) and not of MDPI and/or the editor(s). MDPI and/or the editor(s) disclaim responsibility for any injury to people or property resulting from any ideas, methods, instructions or products referred to in the content.

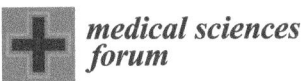

Proceeding Paper

Antibiotic Amnesty: Engaging with the Public across the Midlands Region of England [†]

Rakhi Aggarwal [1,*], Angela Barker [1], Conor Jamieson [2] and Donna Cooper [3]

1. NHS Birmingham and Solihull Integrated Care Board, Birmingham B4 6AR, UK
2. NHS England, Birmingham B2 4BH, UK
3. NHS Black Country Integrated Care Board, Wolverhampton WV1 1SH, UK
* Correspondence: rakhi.aggarwal@nhs.net
† Presented at the 6th Antibiotic Guardian Shared Learning and Awards, Antibiotic Guardian, 2 May 2023; Available online: https://antibioticguardian.com/antibiotic-guardian-2022-shared-learning-awards/.

Abstract: Antimicrobial resistance (AMR) is a major public health threat. The hoarding, sharing and unsafe disposal of unused or expired antibiotics in domestic waste streams or sewage systems by patients may contribute to the risk of acquiring or spreading antibiotic-resistant bacteria. Community pharmacies in the UK accept returned medicines for safe disposal, including antibiotics, but awareness of this is low. We organised an antibiotic amnesty campaign in the Midlands region of England; the aim of the campaign was to raise awareness of the risks of AMR and highlight the safe disposal of antibiotics via community pharmacy, timed to coincide with World Antimicrobial Awareness Week in November 2021.

Keywords: antimicrobial resistance; antibiotic; antibiotic amnesty; community pharmacy; antimicrobial stewardship; awareness

1. Project Overview

An Antibiotic Amnesty campaign for use across the Midlands was developed collaboratively by NHS organisations with Birmingham, Solihull and the Black Country, alongside members of the NHS England regional team. To engage the public locally, the amnesty was actively promoted via the lead Clinical Commissioning Groups (CCGs) involved, GP practices and participating community pharmacies using social media, website content and posters. Community pharmacy teams were invited to participate, with information on the campaign provided via an educational webinar and campaign resources were made available digitally.

The amnesty resource pack included resources in 13 languages and was made available for use across the Midlands, examples are shown in Figure S1. Participating pharmacies promoted the amnesty using the resources provided and had 'amnesty conversations' with the public about the appropriate use of antibiotics. Voluntary data collection by pharmacy teams took place from 15 to 30 November 2021 and included the number of parts or full packs of antibiotics returned, use of the TARGET antibiotic checklist [1] (linking in with the Pharmacy Quality Scheme [2]) and the number of 'amnesty conversations' held. The Local Pharmaceutical Committee (LPC) and Local Authority (LA) collaborated to provide support for the implementation of the project.

2. Outcomes and Impact

The main impact of the campaign was through public engagement, providing an important antimicrobial stewardship (AMS) public health message. Over 7800 members of the public were conversed with, raising awareness of the threat of AMR in addition to the appropriate use of and the safe disposal of antibiotics (Table 1).

Table 1. Outcomes from the community pharmacy based antibiotic amnesty campaign.

Outcome	Number
'Amnesty conversations' with patients and public during the amnesty campaign	7846
TARGET antibiotic checklists completed during the amnesty campaign	4600
Number of full packs of antibiotics returned	126
Number of part packs of antibiotics returned	369

Secondly, there were just under 500 packs or part packs of antibiotics returned for safe disposal. This prevented potentially unsafe disposal of antibiotics, for example, down toilets, sinks or in domestic refuse, and subsequent contamination of the environment. The amnesty also reduced the possibilities of people saving antibiotics for later or sharing them with others, and the subsequent consequences on health and AMR from this.

The final impact of the campaign was the greater collaboration of organisations across the local systems. The development and delivery of the campaign saw collaboration with and engagement from 240 community pharmacy teams, local commissioning and provider organisations, the NHS England regional team, Local Authority, Local Pharmaceutical Committees and other key stakeholders.

3. Future Development

Future development of this campaign involves building on the success of and lessons learned from the 2021 campaign. The aim of future developments will be to increase public engagement by enlisting the support of a wider group of organisations to advertise the campaign to both staff and members of the public. We also plan to include dental surgeries, local NHS Trusts, local universities and local veterinary practices in promoting the campaign; by collaborating with the latter, we aim to include pet owners in the campaign.

We plan to work with local universities to develop and implement pharmacy undergraduate student projects to gather more detail about returned antibiotics. We also plan to trial a public survey using QR codes to gather more qualitative information on patient engagement, attitudes and beliefs about AMR and the impact of the campaign. More considered data collection criteria will enable us to better understand public behaviour around antibiotics and evaluate the campaign more thoroughly.

Furthermore, we hope to develop a post-campaign feedback survey for community pharmacies, to understand their thoughts on what aspects of the campaign could be improved and which went well. By collaborating with the Royal Pharmaceutical Society to host and share campaign resources on their website, we hope to enable other organisations to run similar campaigns and share the resources across England, the rest of the United Kingdom and internationally.

Supplementary Materials: The following supporting information can be downloaded at: https://www.mdpi.com/article/10.3390/msf2022015010/s1, Figure S1: Examples of resources provided for promotion the campaign; Conference Poster: Antibiotic Amnesty: Engaging with the public across the Midlands region of England.

Author Contributions: Conceptualization, R.A., D.C. and C.J.; methodology, R.A., A.B., D.C. and C.J.; formal analysis, R.A., A.B., D.C. and C.J.; investigation, C.J.; resources, R.A., A.B. and C.J.; writing—original draft preparation, R.A., A.B. and C.J.; writing—review and editing, R.A., A.B., D.C. and C.J.; visualization, R.A. and C.J.; supervision, R.A., D.C. and C.J.; project administration, R.A., A.B., D.C. and C.J.; funding acquisition, R.A. and C.J. All authors have read and agreed to the published version of the manuscript.

Funding: This research received no external funding.

Institutional Review Board Statement: Not applicable.

Informed Consent Statement: Not applicable.

Data Availability Statement: The data presented in this study are available on request from the corresponding author. The full data are not publicly available due to the privacy of stakeholders.

Acknowledgments: With thanks to M. Ercolani, J. Dhansey, NHS England Pharmacy Advisors, local pharmaceutical committees and participating pharmacies in the Midlands region, UK Health Security Agency, Local Health Authorities.

Conflicts of Interest: The authors declare no conflict of interest.

References

1. Resources for the Community Pharmacy Setting. Available online: https://elearning.rcgp.org.uk/mod/book/view.php?id=13511&chapterid=784 (accessed on 14 December 2022).
2. Pharmacy Quality Scheme (PQS) 2021/22. Available online: https://www.nhsbsa.nhs.uk/pharmacy-quality-scheme-pqs-202122 (accessed on 14 December 2022).

Disclaimer/Publisher's Note: The statements, opinions and data contained in all publications are solely those of the individual author(s) and contributor(s) and not of MDPI and/or the editor(s). MDPI and/or the editor(s) disclaim responsibility for any injury to people or property resulting from any ideas, methods, instructions or products referred to in the content.

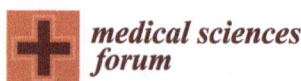

Proceeding Paper

Dental Antimicrobial Prescribing in the Midlands: A Regional Action Plan †

Shima Chundoo [1,*], Conor Jamieson [2], Rob Tobin [3] and Anna Hunt [4]

1. Regional Leadership Fellow, Royal Wolverhampton Hospitals NHS Trust, Wolverhampton WV10 0QP, UK
2. Regional Antimicrobial Stewardship Lead, NHS England, Birmingham B2 4BH, UK
3. Urgent Care Managed Clinical Network West Midlands, Primary Care, Birmingham B37 7TR, UK
4. Dental Public Health, NHS England, Birmingham B2 4BH, UK
* Correspondence: s.chundoo1@nhs.net
† Presented at the 6th Antibiotic Guardian Shared Learning and Awards, Antibiotic Guardian, 2 May 2023; Available online: https://antibioticguardian.com/antibiotic-guardian-2022-shared-learning-awards/.

Abstract: The aim of our project was to create a resource to support an improvement in dental antibiotic prescribing. The initial phase considered antimicrobial prescribing activity, through NHSBSA data collection, which demonstrated that prescribing in the Midlands was higher than the England average. The second phase involved a targeted action plan through the creation of a bespoke regional website. It is a single resource combining the latest evidence-based guidance to tackle inappropriate prescribing and antimicrobial resistance. The national toolkit on Dental Antimicrobial Stewardship was updated for the Midlands, including adapted audit tools. Communication tools were developed, involving patient discussion tools and a multi-professional awareness campaign.

Keywords: dentistry; antimicrobial; antibiotic; antimicrobial resistance; website; governance; audit

Citation: Chundoo, S.; Jamieson, C.; Tobin, R.; Hunt, A. Dental Antimicrobial Prescribing in the Midlands: A Regional Action Plan. *Med. Sci. Forum* **2022**, *15*, 11. https://doi.org/10.3390/msf2022015011

Academic Editor: Diane Ashiru-Oredope

Published: 24 March 2023

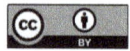

Copyright: © 2023 by the authors. Licensee MDPI, Basel, Switzerland. This article is an open access article distributed under the terms and conditions of the Creative Commons Attribution (CC BY) license (https://creativecommons.org/licenses/by/4.0/).

1. Project Overview

Dental professionals are key stakeholders in tackling antimicrobial resistance (AMR). The UK Government has set tangible targets to tackle AMR as part of the National Action Plan, including to reduce UK antimicrobial use in humans by 15% by 2024 [1]. It has been estimated that primary care dental prescribing accounts for an estimated 7.4% of all antimicrobial prescriptions in England (excluding the private sector and secondary care) [2].

A survey of antimicrobial prescribing amongst dentists in ten English local authorities revealed suboptimal prescribing, including for inappropriate clinical situations and under time pressures [3]. COVID-19 certainly appears to have exacerbated the threat of AMR. Studies appear to suggest that the number of antibiotic prescriptions administered in primary care settings has increased, despite the overall reduced number of appointments [4]. Dental antibiotic prescribing during the pandemic was 20% higher in 2020 compared with the previous year [5]. Antibiotic prescribing increased within the Midlands and was one of the five highest regions within the UK across the pandemic [5].

There are further challenges in regard to the collection of prescribing, or indeed dispensing, data which may not necessarily reflect true prescribing. Overall, there is a lack of appropriate interventions to communicate and target AMR strategies within the Midlands region.

The aim of this project was to create a resource to support an improvement in dental antibiotic prescribing. Further objectives are included to present key prescribing data by different systems. This project comprised two phases. The initial phase considered antimicrobial prescribing activity within the Midlands from data collected by the NHS Business Services Authority (Newcastle Upon Tyne, UK). The results demonstrated that prescribing in the Midlands, particularly the east Midlands, was higher than the England average, as seen in Figure A1. Amoxicillin was the most prescribed antibiotic, as seen in Figure A2. This directly conflicts with recent guidance published by Antimicrobial Prescribing in Dentistry: Good Practice Guidelines, which currently recommends phenoxymethylpenicillin instead of amoxicillin [2].

The second phase involved a targeted regional action plan. Prescribing activity data across the Midlands was presented at local and national meetings by the regional leadership fellow. This permitted an open dialogue with practitioners and key stakeholders, which was enhanced through anonymous feedback and polls. It also enabled a targeted discussion, using tangible figures, to raise awareness. These discussions crystallised the need for a single resource that practitioners can easily refer to for up-to-date guidance and support.

The regional leadership fellow created a bespoke website dedicated to AMR in dentistry. It was designed for patients, the public, professionals and practices. It is a novel single resource combining the latest evidence-based guidance and information to tackle inappropriate prescribing and AMR within dentistry. It is freely accessible through mobile and desktop formats.

Upon centralising antibiotic stewardship information, there was a noted lack of recent updates on the national dental antimicrobial stewardship website, with historic links and new resources missing from the information. The regional leadership fellow updated the national toolkit on Dental Antimicrobial Stewardship to incorporate recently published antimicrobial guidance and new e-learning resources. Audit is a critical step in stewardship, and it provides practitioners with tangible figures on individual practice, which can then be used to drive changes to lead to an improvement in prescribing activity. The current audit had a lack of uptake with clinicians in our region and the regional leadership fellow sought to improve user engagement by specifically adapting the national audit for regional use within primary and secondary care settings. The audit tool was made easier to navigate through drop-down functions and clearer design. This should enable streamlined use of the audit and improve compliance.

The role of non-clinical staff in facilitating a cohesive antimicrobial stewardship message was very much highlighted, as they are the first frontline staff to communicate with patients suffering from toothache. To address this, additional communication tools were developed by the regional leadership fellow. Firstly, a patient discussion tool to assist non-clinical staff when dealing with difficult antibiotic conversations was created, whilst safe-guarding patient care. Secondly, a professional awareness campaign which displays the key aspects of stewardship and how to make an antibiotic pledge was developed. It can be used through a variety of formats (screensaver, poster or printout) for a range of staff members.

2. Outcomes and Impact

2.1. Regional Website Creation

There is a bespoke single-resource website dedicated to tackling AMR and stewardship, which is free to access. It is designed for patients and professionals alike. It covers several domains including stewardship and audit, with the latest links to learning modules and guidance. Further domains are planned, including common infections and additional signposting.

Meaningful engagement is critical to demonstrate that our community is actively engaging with our regional plan and using the latest resources/toolkits to improve practices. Google Analytics are enabled on the website and will be used to continually monitor/track engagement. Although website hits may not necessarily demonstrate direct behaviour change, it is hoped that Google Analytics will demonstrate a measured change in regional engagement with antimicrobial resistance initiatives through website hits. Ultimately, website engagement will demonstrate proof of concept and our regional development.

2.2. Updated Audit Tools

The national audit tool was updated for use within the Midlands and within primary and secondary care settings. Microsoft Excel was used to simplify the audit spreadsheet, with the addition of drop-down functions, which should reduce the time taken to input data. The clearer design and drop-down functions should be easier to navigate and ultimately enable improved compliance with our recommendations. This will enable practices to submit their audits for further incentives, including social media publicity and awards, which will further help to spotlight good practice.

2.3. Communicational Tools

Firstly, a patient discussion tool was created to assist non-clinical staff when dealing with difficult antibiotic conversations, whilst safe-guarding patient care. It is vital that frontline team members are supported in having AMR discussions, with a simple three-step strategy. Secondly, a professional awareness campaign was developed which displays the key aspects of stewardship and how to make an antibiotic pledge. It should help to signpost stakeholders whilst demonstrating engagement.

We plan to review the outcomes of our three key initiatives over a period of 1 year. A range of measured outcomes are planned, including measuring prescribing activity, audit submission and website hits through Google Analytics, (Google 2023, online).

3. Future Development

There are a number of possibilities for our regional project. Firstly, the website is growing, with additional domains planned to further support antibiotic prescribing and tackle AMR. Ongoing updates are planned to ensure that links, communication and interaction with our website are maintained. It is vital to ensure that our website continues to meet the needs of our region. However, we recognise that, long-term, the website will look to be hosted as part of the NHS England website. Google Analytics will be used to monitor and track engagement within our regional action plan. As a region, we believe that a single resource for professionals and the public on dental antimicrobial stewardship and resistance is a fantastic opportunity to reach a wide audience and emphasise a clear message.

Secondly, we recognise the importance of engaging our interprofessional colleagues to assist when patients present with dental infection/conditions. As such, we plan to incorporate an updated list of urgent care practitioners and out-of-hour practices to further signpost on our website. We believe that early intervention and collaboration is key to developing a sustainable long-term plan for tackling antimicrobial resistance. We aim to foster deep connections with adjacent colleagues to promote and support all team members involved in dental prescribing and patient management. As such, dental infection guidance and emergency care signposting have been planned with pharmacy undergraduates at Aston University to further develop interprofessional understanding and contribute to our shared goal. Ultimately, we plan to extend this package towards multi-professional resources and webinars to assist with our regional plan. This will enable a cohesive, multi-professional and collaborative approach to AMR for the future.

Thirdly, we plan to drive regional engagement further by tackling regions with high prescribing activity. Additional meetings and data presentations are planned to further highlight differences in prescribing activity and support practitioners to become more compliant. Practices will be encouraged to submit audit results for further incentives, such as AMR Champion of the Month and social media publicity.

The website and project will continue to develop our website further and engage our region through additional input from the incoming clinical fellow and local Dental Chairs. Ultimately, the aim of our resources is to improve antibiotic prescribing. We hope that by centralising information into a single resource, which is free to access and houses several domains and tools, our regional practitioners will be successful in improving their prescribing activity and tackling AMR.

Supplementary Materials: The following supporting information can be downloaded at: https://www.mdpi.com/article/10.3390/msf2022015011/s1, Conference Poster: Dental Antimicrobial Prescribing in the Midlands: A Regional Action Plan.

Author Contributions: Conceptualization, S.C., C.J. and A.H.; methodology, S.C., C.J. and A.H.; writing—original draft preparation, S.C.; writing—review and editing, S.C., C.J., A.H. and R.T.; supervision, C.J. and A.H.; funding acquisition, S.C. All authors have read and agreed to the published version of the manuscript.

Funding: The website creation, as part of this project, was funded by the Local Dental Network of Birmingham and Solihull.

Institutional Review Board Statement: Not applicable.

Informed Consent Statement: Not applicable.

Data Availability Statement: The data presented in this study are due to become openly available in the NHS Business Services Authority. These data, when available, can be found here: https://www.nhsbsa.nhs.uk/data-release-calendar.

Acknowledgments: We would like to thank Adam Morby, Regional Chief Dentist, for his support and guidance throughout this project. We would like to kindly thank Elizabeth Beech and the NHSBSA for dispensing data provision. We would also like to kindly thank Peter Thornley, Local Dental Network Chair of Birmingham and Solihull, for his support and provision of funding towards the website.

Conflicts of Interest: The authors declare no conflict of interest. The funders had no role in the design of the study; in the collection, analyses, or interpretation of data; in the writing of the manuscript; or in the decision to publish the results.

Appendix A

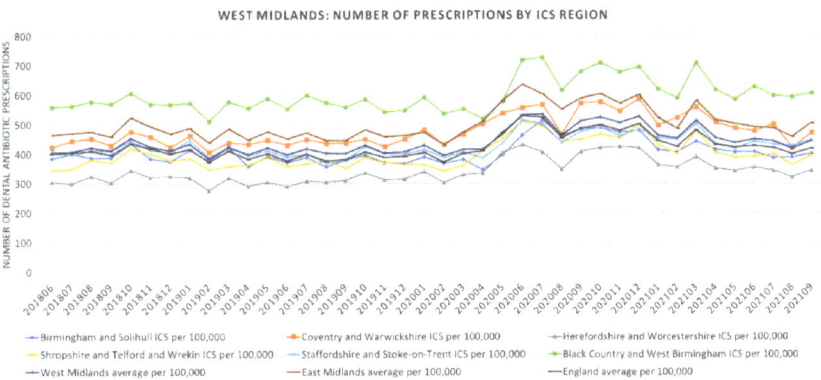

Figure A1. Number of prescriptions in the west Midlands per 100,000, by integrated care systems, and using ONS mid-year population estimates.

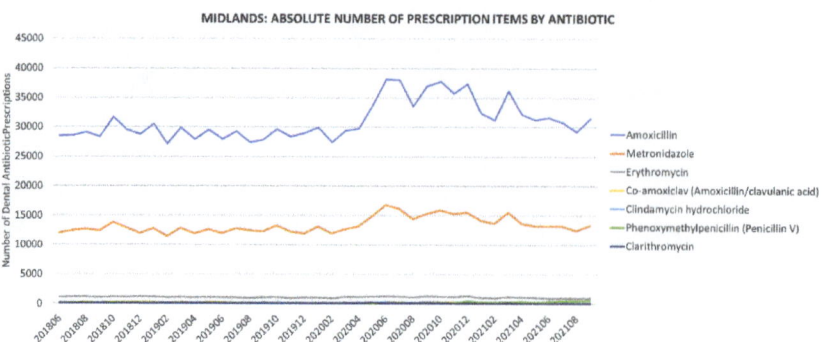

Figure A2. Absolute number of prescription items by antibiotic in the Midlands.

References

1. Tackling Antimicrobial Resistance 2019–2024: The UK's Five-Year National Action Plan. Available online: https://assets.publishing.service.gov.uk/government/uploads/system/uploads/attachment_data/file/1070263/UK_AMR_5_year_national_action_plan.pdf (accessed on 8 August 2022).
2. Palmer, N. (Ed.) *Antimicrobial Prescribing in Dentistry: Good Practice Guidelines*, 3rd ed.; Faculty of General Dental Practice (UK) and Faculty of Dental Surgery: London, UK, 2020.
3. Palmer, N.A.O.; Pealing, R.; Ireland, R.S.; Martin, M.V. A study of therapeutic antibiotic prescribing in National Health Service general dental practice in England. *Br. Dent. J.* **2000**, *188*, 554–558. [CrossRef] [PubMed]
4. Armitage, R.; Nellums, L.B. Antibiotic prescribing in general practice during COVID-19. *Lancet Infect. Dis.* **2020**, *21*, e144. [CrossRef] [PubMed]
5. Shah, S.; Wordley, V.; Thompson, W. How did COVID-19 impact on dental antibiotic prescribing across England? *Br. Dent. J.* **2020**, *229*, 601–604. [CrossRef] [PubMed]

Disclaimer/Publisher's Note: The statements, opinions and data contained in all publications are solely those of the individual author(s) and contributor(s) and not of MDPI and/or the editor(s). MDPI and/or the editor(s) disclaim responsibility for any injury to people or property resulting from any ideas, methods, instructions or products referred to in the content.

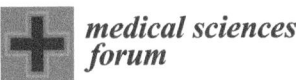 *medical sciences forum*

Proceeding Paper

Development and User Feedback on Antimicrobial Stewardship Explainer Videos: A Collaborative Approach between the UK and Eight African Countries [†]

Jessica Fraser [1,*], Frances Garraghan [2,3] and Diane Ashiru-Oredope [2,4]

1. Tropical Health and Education Trust, London EC2A 4NE, UK
2. Commonwealth Pharmacists Association, London E1W 1AW, UK
3. Manchester University NHS Foundation Trust, Manchester M13 9WL, UK
4. Pharmaceutical Public Health Department, University of Nottingham, Nottingham NG7 2RD, UK

* Correspondence: jessica.fraser@thet.org
† Presented at the 6th Antibiotic Guardian Shared Learning and Awards, Antibiotic Guardian, 2 May 2023; Available online: https://antibioticguardian.com/antibiotic-guardian-2022-shared-learning-awards/

Abstract: Antimicrobial resistance is a growing, complex, and global threat. Health partnerships are working to address antimicrobial resistance through antimicrobial stewardship activities. To support this work, the Commonwealth Partnerships for Antimicrobial Stewardship programme developed four antimicrobial stewardship explainer animation videos in eight different accents, with input from over 50 stakeholders across eight African countries and the UK. The videos highlight different scenarios and explain AMS in easy-to-understand ways for both health practitioners and the public. Health partnerships piloted the videos in several ways, including in clinical waiting rooms, trainings, and AMS meetings, and provided feedback in a survey. In total, 94% of survey respondents gave the videos either a '5' or '4' for usefulness, with '5' indicating 'very useful'. Moving forward, through collaboration with the health partnerships, the videos will continue to be disseminated and adapted.

Keywords: antimicrobial resistance; antimicrobial stewardship; health partnerships; explainer videos

---

Citation: Fraser, J.; Garraghan, F.; Ashiru-Oredope, D. Development and User Feedback on Antimicrobial Stewardship Explainer Videos: A Collaborative Approach between the UK and Eight African Countries. *Med. Sci. Forum* **2022**, *15*, 15. https://doi.org/10.3390/msf2022015015

Academic Editor: Jordan Charlesworth

Published: 28 March 2023

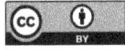

Copyright: © 2022 by the authors. Licensee MDPI, Basel, Switzerland. This article is an open access article distributed under the terms and conditions of the Creative Commons Attribution (CC BY) license (https://creativecommons.org/licenses/by/4.0/).

1. Project Overview

Background: Antimicrobial resistance (AMR) is a growing, complex, and global threat. Many factors have accelerated its spread, including overuse and misuse of medicines in humans, livestock, and agriculture, as well as poor access to clean water, poor sanitation, and poor hygiene [1]. Across Africa, AMR is particularly concerning and the impact is becoming more apparent, with healthcare-associated infections increasing, the ongoing high burden of communicable diseases, and weak and fragmented public and animal health systems [1,2]. Health partnerships are working to address AMR through antimicrobial stewardship (AMS), infection prevention and control (IPC), and developing pharmacy expertise and capacity.

The videos: To support AMS, the Tropical Health and Education Trust (THET) and the Commonwealth Pharmacists Association (CPA, as part of the Commonwealth Partnerships for the Antimicrobial Stewardship (CwPAMS) scheme, with funding from the Fleming Fund and input from more than 50 stakeholders across the UK and eight African countries, developed four AMS explainer animation videos with the video animation company Video Symmetry. The videos present different situations, stories, and information to help explain AMS in easy-to-understand ways.

The audience: the videos are designed for both the public and health practitioners.

Process of development: From 2021 to 2022, key stakeholders were engaged from a range of backgrounds and experience, including healthcare informants and external advisers (e.g., the Africa Centres for Disease Control and WHO). A brainstorming stakeholder workshop was held to determine the scope of the videos. The workshop concluded that English was the most useful language for the videos, but different accents were recorded so the characters could be relatable in multiple contexts. Scripts were developed through several iterations and reviewing sessions with stakeholders. Draft storyboard animations were developed by Video Symmetry and shared with the reviewers for further feedback on clinical accuracy, appropriateness, and ease of understanding. Several review phases were necessary to ensure that the videos were both technically and contextually accurate and appropriate. The main challenge was to make the complexity of AMS/AMR easily understandable to a wide audience. Following the completion of priority edits, three of the four videos were uploaded to YouTube and shared with the health partnerships to pilot in training sessions during May 2022. A feedback survey was shared with the partnerships to inform on the use, value, and next steps for the videos.

2. Outcomes and Impact

Outcome: Following the development process, four video topics were confirmed. As a result, the videos cover the following topics:

1. The patient and doctor experience with antimicrobials. This video explores a mother and father's experience with seeking medical help for their child's illness, such as learning when it is appropriate to use antimicrobials or not, and the preventative actions one can take to reduce the chances of AMR.
2. Continuum of care. This video explores the different roles involved in the whole journey of care. For example, for the doctor, the journey is about carrying out the appropriate test or using relevant tools/guidelines to assess the patient; for the pharmacist, providing advice to colleagues and dispensing the correct antimicrobials; for the nurse, providing the antibiotic on time and appropriately; and for the patient, taking the medicine correctly and not sharing antimicrobials with family, friends, or pets.
3. Surgical prophylaxis. This video explores the journey of healthcare professionals (doctor, nurse, and pharmacist) in managing surgical-site infection, using the WHO Surgical Safety Checklist, and deciding on the appropriate use of antimicrobials in a patient's journey to reduce the risk of AMR.
4. Defining AMR and AMS. This video defines antimicrobial resistance and stewardship, reviews the global organisations involved in AMR prevention, assesses why it is important that we tackle it, and determines the actions that individuals (both patients and health professionals) can take to reduce AMR.

Impact: From the analysis of the 52 pilot-survey respondents, who were from a range of clinical cadres and civil-society organisations, the videos have demonstrated to be useful and positive for the health partnerships. For example, 49 (94%) survey respondents gave the videos either a '5' or '4' for usefulness, with '5' indicating 'very useful'. Respondents were also asked how they have used the videos thus far in their work. Some examples of responses include:

- Training workshops involving 50+ and 145+ people;
- Seminars of 20+ people and in AMS team meetings;
- One partnership bought a TV to share the videos with hospital staff/students in the clinical skills training room at the hospital. This room is used for small group teaching sessions;
- One partnership showcased the videos during training sessions and trainees then translated the videos into Swahili for future use.

In addition, respondents were asked how they expect to use the videos in their practice, institutions, and networks in the future; the data gathered for this question are represented in Figure 1.

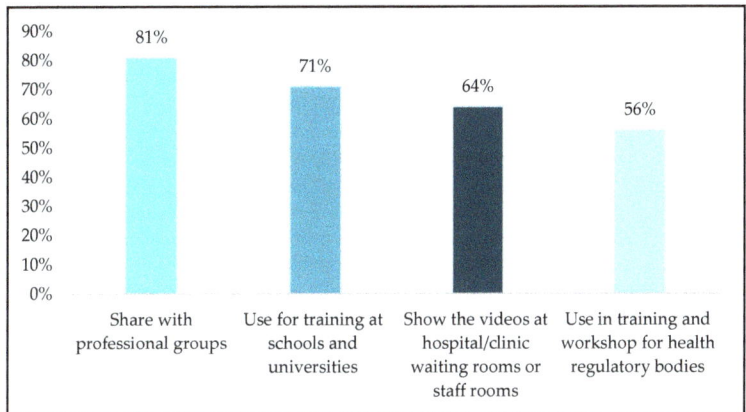

Figure 1. Question addressed: what are the main ways that survey respondents will use the videos?

Lastly, we assessed what respondents learned from the videos. When asked which video they learned from the most, 24 (47%) survey respondents stated they learned the most from the patient-experience video, 19 (37%) from the continuum of care, and 8 (15%) from the surgical prophylaxis. Respondents also provided qualitative feedback on the videos; for example, the feedback included "Get these out there, they are outstanding!", "These are PERFECT for Public Health Promotion programmes", and "Very strong videos-useful for a range of training situations".

3. Future Development

All the videos are now available on YouTube [3]. To further develop and disseminate the videos, we plan to do the following activities:

- Continue to gather feedback from health partnerships and, where feasible, make priority edits to the videos regarding suggestions that were made in the survey. For example, adding more languages, improving existing accents where needed, and providing subtitles with local languages to improve accessibility;
- Disseminate the videos during future phases of the CwPAMS programme and encourage health partnerships to use the videos in training sessions and at the hospitals/clinics;
- Support health partnerships to disseminate the videos on a wider scale. Partnerships have expressed interest in sharing the videos on, for example, TV/radio shows, social media, and through printed screenshots of the videos on posters;
- Share the videos with a wider network of stakeholders, including, for example, the Africa CDC, Fleming Fund, and WHO, to support further antimicrobial stewardship.

Supplementary Materials: The poster is available at https://www.mdpi.com/article/10.3390/msf2022015015/s1, Poster: Development and user feedback on Antimicrobial Stewardship Explainer Videos: a collaborative approach between the UK and eight African countries.

Author Contributions: Conceptualization, F.G., D.A.-O. and J.F.; methodology, F.G., D.A.-O. and J.F.; coordination of videos development and project management, J.F.; review and technical feedback and input, F.G. and D.A.-O.; data curation, J.F.; writing and editing, J.F.; review, F.G. and D.A.-O.; supervision, F.G. and D.A.-O. All authors have read and agreed to the published version of the manuscript.

Funding: This research received no external funding.

Institutional Review Board Statement: Not applicable.

Informed Consent Statement: Not applicable.

Data Availability Statement: Data available on request due to privacy restrictions. The data presented in this study are available on request from the corresponding author. The data are not publicly available due to organisational details being provided by survey respondents.

Acknowledgments: We would like to thank all the contributors from the nine countries for all their time, input, and expertise for these videos. This project was part of the Commonwealth Partnerships for Antimicrobial Stewardship (CwPAMS), managed by the Tropical Health and Education Trust (THET) and Commonwealth Pharmacists Association (CPA). CwPAMS is funded by the Fleming Fund using UK aid-funding. The Fund is managed by the UK Department of Health and Social Care and invests in strengthening surveillance systems through a portfolio of country and regional grants, global projects and fellowship schemes. The views expressed in this publication are those of the authors and not necessarily those of the UK Department of Health and Social Care, the NHS, the represented NHS Trusts, CPA, or THET.

Conflicts of Interest: The authors declare no conflict of interest.

References

1. Fraser, J.L.; Alimi, Y.H.; Varma, J.K.; Muraya, T.; Kujinga, T.; Carter, V.K.; Schultsz, C.; Del Rio Vilas, V.J. Antimicrobial resistance control efforts in Africa: A survey of the role of Civil Society Organisations. *Glob. Health Action* **2021**, *14*, 1868055. [CrossRef] [PubMed]
2. Varma, J.K.; Oppong-Otoo, J.; Ondoa, P.; Perovic, O.; Park, B.J.; Laxminarayan, R.; Peeling, R.W.; Schultsz, C.; Li, H.; Ihekweazu, C.; et al. Africa Centres for Disease Control and Prevention's framework for antimicrobial resistance control in Africa. *Afr. J. Lab. Med.* **2018**, *7*, 830. [CrossRef] [PubMed]
3. AMS Explainer Animation Videos–Pilot. THET Partnerships YouTube. Available online: https://youtube.com/playlist?list=PL9qDtywmdsRBhwyc0XFUz5204Z1vQCrWd (accessed on 15 August 2022).

Disclaimer/Publisher's Note: The statements, opinions and data contained in all publications are solely those of the individual author(s) and contributor(s) and not of MDPI and/or the editor(s). MDPI and/or the editor(s) disclaim responsibility for any injury to people or property resulting from any ideas, methods, instructions or products referred to in the content.

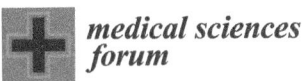

Proceeding Paper

Schoolchildren as Agents of Change towards Antimicrobial Resistance [†]

Michael Mosha [1,*], Erick Venant [1], Baltazari Stanley [1], Fatuma Denis [1], Dorinegrace Mushi [1], Eva Ombaka [2] and Karin Wiedenmayer [3,4]

1. Roll Back Antimicrobial Resistance Initiative, Dodoma P.O. Box 2125, Tanzania
2. Faculty of Pharmaceutics, St. John's University of Tanzania, Dodoma P.O. Box 47, Tanzania
3. Swiss Tropical and Public Health Institute, P.O. Box, CH-4123, Allschwil, Switzerland
4. University of Basel, P.O. Box, CH-4003 Basel, Switzerland
* Correspondence: michaelmosha@rbainitiative.or.tz; Tel.: +255-659752233
† Presented at the 6th Antibiotic Guardian Shared Learning and Awards, Antibiotic Guardian, 2 May 2023; Available online: https://antibioticguardian.com/antibiotic-guardian-2022-shared-learning-awards/.

Abstract: Schoolchildren are in their formative years, and therefore at an ideal stage in their lives to take in knowledge and best practices that will guide their future behavior. Through the Roll Back Antimicrobial Resistance (RBA) Initiative in Tanzania, antimicrobial resistance (AMR) School Clubs have successfully educated and empowered schoolchildren to become antibiotic guardians and AMR champions. Using appropriate language and consideration of the local context, the project has employed a variety of innovative activities, including AMR arts and crafts, competitions, storytelling and interactive learning that would teach children in an engaging and enjoyable manner. The School Club project has demonstrated how a mix of fun-based knowledge and skills transfer methods and rewarding competitions can change antimicrobial use knowledge and practice in schoolchildren.

Keywords: antimicrobial resistance; RBA Initiative; AMR School Clubs; schoolchildren

1. Project Overview

Antimicrobial resistance (AMR) refers to the ability of infectious microorganisms to resist medicines [1] and is primarily caused by the misuse of medicines [2]. Educating people on the basic knowledge and best practices in the use of medicines, at an early stage in their lives, may positively shape the behavior of a future patient population. Schoolchildren are in their formative years, and therefore at an optimal stage in their lives to take in knowledge and best practices that will guide their own behavior. Moreover, as they are connected with families, communities and are future leaders and healthcare providers, they may exert a positive impact within their networks. The Roll Back Antimicrobial Resistance (RBA) Initiative is a registered non–governmental organization in Tanzania that aims to fight back AMR. The organization sees both rural and urban communities as critical players in addressing AMR. The RBA Initiative promotes the rational use of antimicrobials, conducts research on AMR, facilitates dissemination of knowledge on AMR and promotes behavioral change, with the aim of reducing the rate of infection due to AMR. The Initiative has been pioneering work with young people as agents of change to increase AMR awareness and to promote positive behavioral changes.

The RBA Initiative has implemented the AMR School Clubs project in the Dodoma region in Tanzania. The project consists of educating and empowering schoolchildren in selected schools to become agents of change who, in turn, will encourage the community to adopt positive behaviors that will prevent the spread and emergency of AMR.

The project also sensitizes on the "One Health" approach [3] as a key tool to contain AMR. The RBA Initiative uses different strategies to enhance understanding of AMR while encouraging creativity and innovation among the students. Using appropriate language and consideration of the local context, the project employs a variety of innovative activities, including AMR arts and crafts (i.e., songs, drama, traditional dance, drawing and poems), competitions, storytelling and interactive learning as a set of fun activities, integrated with classroom teaching [4].

The main objective is to equip schoolchildren with the knowledge and skills to understand antimicrobial use and AMR and with the ability to pass the knowledge to their families, other students and the community at large.

2. Results and Outcomes

Through the RBA Initiative, AMR School Clubs have successfully educated and empowered schoolchildren to become antibiotic guardians and AMR champions. The RBA Initiative has reached 11,552 schoolchildren from 25 Tanzanian schools, including primary and secondary schools [5].

The organization also commissioned a hand washing station and water tank to a secondary school, dedicated to the AMR arts and crafts competition winner. This allows educating schoolchildren about hand hygiene.

Students who have completed training, but have moved to other schools in various regions to pursue further studies, are supported and guided to continue spreading key AMR messages as AMR champions in their new communities and schools. A selection of stories of some of the AMR champions is accessible via: https://rbainitiative.or.tz/events.php (accessed on 22 November 2022).

Rhoda, a 15-year-old student, shared her story of how the education she has received in the AMR School Club has transformed her own life and that of her community. She said, "Attending an AMR Club has made a huge difference in my life. I have learned so many things, like the importance of hand-washing and hygiene, how to identify fake medicine and the importance of always completing the full course of antibiotics (even after feeling well). I've also learned that we should never share our medicine with anyone". Rhoda's account captures the voice and experience of many schoolchildren in Tanzania. The full story is accessible via: https://www.stopsuperbugs.co.uk/stories/story/Rhodas-story/ (accessed on 22 November 2022).

The arts and crafts work, such as songs and dramas composed by the RBA Initiative and AMR Club members, can successfully be used as educational entertainment, for instance using the YouTube channel.

The RBA Initiative has increased the AMR knowledge of School Club members. In an interventional pre-post comparative study, data were collected before and after training on antimicrobial use and resistance. Three aspects were investigated: (i) awareness of ways to reduce AMR; (ii) knowledge that antibiotics cannot be used to treat flu; and (iii) factors that contribute to AMR. Before the training, knowledge of these aspects was below 37%. Three months after the training, average knowledge had increased to above 90% [3].

The head of Mkonze Secondary School, Mr. Andrew Rumishael, explained how the RBA Initiative's AMR School Clubs project is making a positive change, not only through AMR education, but also through improving WASH infrastructure and hand hygiene. "We are very grateful for the handwashing station. This station is a great help for current and future schoolchildren with hand hygiene. We have not only benefited from AMR education, but also the WASH infrastructure". He further explained how AMR education, provided through this project, benefited the community and the family members through trained students. Mr. Andrew Rumishael's account is accessible via: https://www.youtube.com/watch?v=7hwOeXcTxCc (accessed on 22 November 2022).

The RBA Initiative AMR School Club project has demonstrated how a mix of fun-based knowledge and skills transfer and rewarding competitions can change antimicrobial use knowledge and practice in schoolchildren. During the United Nations AMR-High-level Interactive Dialogue, the RBA Initiative AMR School Clubs project was cited as an important example of creative, community-focused support [4,6].

3. Future Development

In order to reach more schoolchildren across a wider geographic area in Tanzania, the RBA Initiative keeps seeking financial support to scale up the AMR School Clubs. The organization intends to utilize the lessons learned by engaging the trained students who are AMR champions to continue acting as agents of change in their communities. As part of sharing best practices and exploring how this approach could be applied in other countries, the RBA Initiative is proactively disseminating its project outcomes and findings to a broader audience at various conferences and meetings.

Author Contributions: Conceptualization, M.M. and E.V.; methodology B.S.; investigation D.M.; resources F.D.; draft preparation, M.M. and E.V.; review and editing, E.V., K.W. and E.O.; project administration, F.D. All authors have read and agreed to the published version of the manuscript.

Funding: This research received no external funding, but the APC was funded by Antibiotic Guardian Shared Learning Event and Awards.

Institutional Review Board Statement: Not applicable.

Informed Consent Statement: Informed consent was obtained from all subjects involved in the study.

Data Availability Statement: No new data were created or analyzed in this study. Data sharing is not applicable to this article.

Acknowledgments: We acknowledge the financial and material support offered by the Queen's Common Trust and British Society of Antimicrobial Chemotherapy, respectively, and also the administrative and technical support offered by the RBA Initiative team.

Conflicts of Interest: The authors declare no conflict of interest.

References

1. Simonsen, G.S.; Tapsall, J.W.; Allegranzi, B.; Talbot, E.A.; Lazzari, S. The antimicrobial resistance containment and surveillance approach-a public health tool. *Bull. World Health Organ.* **2004**, *82*, 928–934. [PubMed]
2. Horumpende, P.G.; Sonda, T.B.; van Zwetselaar, M.; Antony, M.L.; Tenu, F.F.; Mwanziva, C.E.; Shao, E.R.; Mshana, S.E.; Mmbaga, B.T.; Chilongola, J.O. Prescription and non-prescription antibiotic dispensing practices in part I and part II pharmacies in Moshi Municipality, Kilimanjaro Region in Tanzania: A simulated clients approach. *PLoS ONE* **2018**, *13*, e0207465. [CrossRef] [PubMed]
3. WHO. *A One Health Priority Research Agenda for Antimicrobial Resistance*; WHO: Geneva, Switzerland, 2023.
4. Venant, E.; Stanley, B.K.; Mosha, M.J.; Mushi, D.J.; Masanja, P.; Wiedenmayer, K.; Ombaka, E. Assessment of knowledge, attitude and practice towards antimicrobial use and resistance among students in three secondary schools in dodoma city. *JAC Antimicrob. Resist.* **2022**, *4*, i14. [CrossRef]
5. RBA Initiative Annual Report 2021–2022. Available online: https://rbainitiative.or.tz/pdf/RBAI-ANNUAL-REPORT-2021-2022.pdf (accessed on 22 November 2022).
6. UN AMR-High-Level Interactive Dialogue, UN General Assembly. Available online: https://www.youtube.com/watch?v=v_auNJmjNEI (accessed on 22 November 2022).

Disclaimer/Publisher's Note: The statements, opinions and data contained in all publications are solely those of the individual author(s) and contributor(s) and not of MDPI and/or the editor(s). MDPI and/or the editor(s) disclaim responsibility for any injury to people or property resulting from any ideas, methods, instructions or products referred to in the content.

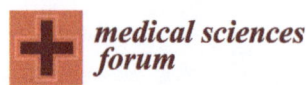 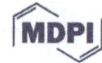

Editorial

Statement of Peer Review [†]

Diane Ashiru-Oredope *, Carry Triggs-Hodge and Jordan Charlesworth

HCAI, Fungal, AMR, AMU & Sepsis Division, UK Health Security Agency, London SW1P 3JR, UK; carry.triggshodge@ukhsa.gov.uk (C.T.-H.); jordan.charlesworth@ukhsa.gov.uk (J.C.)
* Correspondence: diane.ashiru-oredope@ukhsa.gov.uk
† Presented at the ESPAUR 2021/22 Webinar, Antibiotic Guardian, 23 November 2022; Available online: https://antibioticguardian.com/Meetings/espaur-2021-22-webinar/, or presented at the 6th Antibiotic Guardian Shared Learning and Awards, Antibiotic Guardian, 2 May 2023; Available online: https://antibioticguardian.com/antibiotic-guardian-2022-shared-learning-awards/.

In submitting conference proceedings to *Medical Sciences Forum*, the volume editors of the proceedings certify to the publisher that all papers published in this volume have been subjected to peer review administered by the volume editors. Reviews were conducted by expert referees to the professional and scientific standards expected of a proceedings journal.

- Type of peer review: single-blind.
- Conference submission management system: email.
- Number of submissions sent for review: 9 (ESPAUR 2021/22 Webinar); 60 (Antibiotic Guardian Awards).
- Number of submissions accepted: 8 (ESPAUR 2021/22 Webinar); 12 (Antibiotic Guardian Awards).
- Number of submissions published: 8 (ESPAUR 2021/22 Webinar); 12 (Antibiotic Guardian Awards).
- Acceptance rate (number of submissions accepted/number of submissions received): 88.9% (ESPAUR 2021/22 Webinar); 20% (Antibiotic Guardian Awards).
- Average number of reviews per paper: 1 (ESPAUR 2021/22 Webinar); 3.5 (Antibiotic Guardian Awards).
- Total number of reviewers involved: 6 (ESPAUR 2021/22 Webinar); 33 (Antibiotic Guardian Awards).
- Any additional information on the review process can be found below.

1. ESPAUR Report Webinar and Antibiotic Guardian Shared Learning Events

The ESPAUR (English Surveillance Programme for Antimicrobial Utilisation and Resistance) national annual report 2021–2022 comprises chapters on Antimicrobial resistance, Antimicrobial consumption, Antimicrobial stewardship, NHS England: improvement and assurance schemes, Professional education, training and public engagement, COVID-19 Therapeutics, Research, and Stakeholder Engagement. The report was published online (https://www.gov.uk/government/publications/english-surveillance-programme-antimicrobial-utilisation-and-resistance-espaur-report (accessed on 24 October 2023)) by UKHSA on 21 November 2022.

UKHSA hosted the ESPAUR 2021-22 Report interactive online webinar on Wednesday 23 November 2022, where a summary of the key findings covering each chapter was presented. Attendees were provided with the opportunity to submit questions prior to the event and during live Q&A sections of the webinar. They were also invited to complete a feedback form after the event. The data were acquired from 1 April 2021 to 31 March 2022. Moreover, the displayed recording and the slide set were uploaded onto the Antibiotic Guardian website (https://antibioticguardian.com/Meetings/espaur-2021-22-webinar/ (accessed on 24 October 2023)).

Citation: Ashiru-Oredope, D.; Triggs-Hodge, C.; Charlesworth, J. Statement of Peer Review. *Med. Sci. Forum* **2023**, *15*, 21. https://doi.org/10.3390/msf2022015021

Published: 3 November 2023

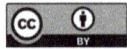

Copyright: © 2023 by the authors. Licensee MDPI, Basel, Switzerland. This article is an open access article distributed under the terms and conditions of the Creative Commons Attribution (CC BY) license (https://creativecommons.org/licenses/by/4.0/).

2. Antibiotic Guardian Shared Learning & Awards Event (AGSLA)

The Antibiotic Guardian Shared Learning and Awards (AGSLA) event was initiated in 2016 to acknowledge, celebrate and share the practical knowledge of healthcare professionals across the UK and abroad in tackling antimicrobial resistance. The 2022/23 AGSLA was opened for entries between 4th July 2022 and 12th September 2022. A total of 60 entries were received across 11 categories, which are summarized below (Table 1).

Table 1. Summarized entries.

Award Category	Number of Judges/Reviewers	Number of Entries	Number Shortlisted
Animal Health	4	4	4
Children & Family	5	1	1
Community Communications	3	5	3
COVID-19 Learning	5	3	3
Diagnostic Stewardship	4	3	2
Innovation & technology	3	6	3
Multi-country collaboration	3	3	2
Prescribing & stewardship	7	18	3
Public Engagement	4	7	5
Research	3	5	3
Das Pillay Antimicrobial Stewardship Memorial Award	4	5	3

Each entry was judged as part of the shortlisting process by a minimum of three independent judges. Judges were asked to declare any conflicts of interests at the point of judging—which they did not score. Submissions were scored out of ten against five categories (originality, engagement, success, impact, and future development), ranging from a low (one) to a high (ten) score.

Entries with sufficiently high scores were eligible to be shortlisted for an award (a total of 32) and were offered the opportunity to adapt their award's entry—based on the judges' peer review comments—before being submitted to the journal. The entrants were asked to adapt their entry's wording (as per the judges' peer review) and submit it via the provided abstract template.

Shortlisting/Judging Panel (Peer Reviewers)

Dr Aaron Brady—Lead Antimicrobial Pharmacist, Belfast Health & Social Care Trust.
Dr Abid Hussain—Consultant Medical Microbiologist, University Hospitals Birmingham.
Ms Amy Jackson—Senior Project Manager, UK Health Security Agency.
Ms Carole Fry—Infection Prevention & Control Lead, UK Health Security Agency.
Mrs Claire Brandish—Anti-Infectives Pharmacist, Buckinghamshire Healthcare NHS Trust.
Dr Conor Jamieson—Regional AMS Lead, NHS England.
Prof Diane Ashiru-Oredope—National Lead, Antibiotic Guardian campaign and WAAW/EAAD planning group (England); Lead Pharmacist, Antimicrobial Resistance Programme, UK Health Security Agency.
Ms Elizabeth Beech—Regional AMS Lead, NHS England.
Ms Ella Casale—Interim TB/AMR Programme Manager, UKHSA East of England; AMR Programme Officer, UK Health Security Agency.
Dr Emma Budd—Senior Scientist (Epidemiology), UK Health Security Agency.
Ms Eno Umoh—Scientific Coordinator, Imperial College London.

Mrs Fran Garraghan—Antimicrobial stewardship pharmacist, Manchester University NHS Foundation Trust.

Ms Fran Husson—Public Partner/Lay Member, English Surveillance Programme for Antimicrobial Utilisation and Resistance.

Prof James Wood—Dean of Cambridge Veterinary School, University of Cambridge.

Mr Jonathan Underhill—Consultant Clinical Adviser—NICE.

Mr Jordan Charlesworth—Programme Manager—COVID-19 Therapeutics Programme, UKHSA.

Dr Julie Robotham—Head of Modelling & Evaluations, UK Health Security Agency.

Ms Katherine Le Bosquet—Lead Pharmacist for Frailty and Elderly Medicine, Medway NHS Foundation Trust.

Dr Lisa Ritchie—Head of Infection Prevention & Control, NHS England.

Dr Louise Dunsmure—Consultant Pharmacist – Antimicrobial Stewardship, Oxford University Hospitals NHS Foundation Trust.

Dr Mariyam Mirfenderesky—Consultant Medical Microbiologist, UK Health Security Agency.

Mr Michael Corley—Head of Policy & Public Affairs, BSAC.

Dr Musarrat Afza—Consultant in Communicable Disease Control, UK Health Security Agency.

Dr Naomi Fleming—Regional AMS Lead, NHS England.

Mr Peter Boriello—Former Chief Executive, Veterinary Medicines Directorate.

Prof Philip Howard—Regional AMS Lead, NHS England.

Ms Preety Ramdut—Regional AMS Lead, NHS England.

Ms Rita Huyton—Nurse Consultant, UK Health Security Agency.

Ms Rosemary Stevenson—Scientific programme lead, NHS England.

Ms Sejal Parekh—Senior Policy Manager, NHS England.

Prof Tracey Thronley—Head of Clinical Research & Outcomes, Boots UK.

Dr William Welfare—Consultant in Health Protection, UK Health Security Agency.

Dr Yvonne Dailey—Consultant in Dental Public Health, UK Health Security Agency.

Conflicts of Interest: The authors declare no conflict of interest.

Disclaimer/Publisher's Note: The statements, opinions and data contained in all publications are solely those of the individual author(s) and contributor(s) and not of MDPI and/or the editor(s). MDPI and/or the editor(s) disclaim responsibility for any injury to people or property resulting from any ideas, methods, instructions or products referred to in the content.

MDPI
St. Alban-Anlage 66
4052 Basel
Switzerland
www.mdpi.com

Medical Sciences Forum Editorial Office
E-mail: msf@mdpi.com
www.mdpi.com/journal/msf

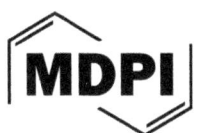

Disclaimer/Publisher's Note: The statements, opinions and data contained in all publications are solely those of the individual author(s) and contributor(s) and not of MDPI and/or the editor(s). MDPI and/or the editor(s) disclaim responsibility for any injury to people or property resulting from any ideas, methods, instructions or products referred to in the content.

www.ingramcontent.com/pod-product-compliance
Lightning Source LLC
LaVergne TN
LVHW070543100526
838202LV00012B/361